DR. LAWRENCE HORNICK
Massapequa Park, New York 11762

Basic Electrocardiography Handbook

Basic Electrocardiography Handbook

Leonard J. Lyon, M.D., F.A.C.P.

Clinical Associate Professor
College of Medicine and Dentistry of New Jersey at Newark

VNR VAN NOSTRAND REINHOLD COMPANY
NEW YORK   CINCINNATI   ATLANTA   DALLAS   SAN FRANCISCO
LONDON   TORONTO   MELBOURNE

Van Nostrand Reinhold Company Regional Offices:
New York   Cincinnati   Atlanta   Dallas   San Francisco

Van Nostrand Reinhold Company International Offices:
London   Toronto   Melbourne

Copyright © 1977 by Litton Educational Publishing, Inc.

Library of Congress Catalog Card Number: 77-8321
ISBN: 0-442-24960-8

All rights reserved. No part of this work covered by the copyright hereon may be reproduced or used in any form or by any means—graphic, electronic, or mechanical, including photo-copying, recording, taping, or information storage and retrieval systems—without permission of the publisher.

Manufactured in the United States of America

Published by Van Nostrand Reinhold Company
450 West 33rd Street, New York, N.Y. 10001

Published simultaneously in Canada by Van Nostrand Reinhold Ltd.

15 14 13 12 11 10 9 8 7 6 5 4 3 2 1

Library of Congress Cataloging in Publication Data

Lyon, Leonard J
   Basic electrocardiography handbook.

   Includes index.
   1. Electrocardiography.   I. Title.
[DNLM: 1. Electrocardiography—Handbooks. WG140
L991b]
RC683.5.E5L9   616.1'2'0754   77-8321
ISBN 0-442-24960-8

For Susan, Eric and Giles

Preface

This book is an outgrowth of several years of formal and informal teaching of electrocardiography to technicians, nurses, medical students and physicians. It is not an encyclopedic text, but one that focuses on acute cardiology. I have tried to make it sufficiently comprehensive to enable the reader to analyze and interpret any electrocardiogram likely to be recorded from a patient with a suddenly developing or potentially life-threatening cardiac disorder.

The main emphasis has been placed on the diagnosis of arrhythmias and conduction disorders, with other sections on myocardial ischemia and infarction, digitalis, pericarditis, pulmonary embolism, potassium problems, preexcitation and pacemakers. However, the interpretation of any electrocardiogram is limited by the quality of the electrocardiogram itself; so, after reviewing basic cardiac anatomy, physiology and electrocardiographic measurements, the first chapter deals with the recognition and correction of common recording errors.

I have deliberately omitted discussion of atrial and ventricular hypertrophy, cardiomyopathies, valvular and congenital heart disease, because immediate electrocardiographic diagnosis is not usually crucial in these conditions. My goal has been to provide the information and skills necessary for on-the-spot electrocardiographic diagnosis of acute or potentially lethal conditions so that appropriate therapy can be promptly initiated, or so that accurate information can be immediately relayed to the responsible physician without the hours to days of delay that may follow when an electrocardiogram goes through "normal channels" for interpretation.

This book would not have been possible without the enthusiastic support of the electrocardiographic technicians and nursing staffs of the Bergen Pines and Pascack Valley Hospitals, the nurses of the Woodcliff Lake Manor Nursing Home and my own office staff, all of whom were more than generous in helping me collect illustrative electrocardiograms. I am also indebted to Claire Seyffer for outstanding secretarial assistance, and, above all, to my family for providing the peace and tranquility I needed for the completion of this project.

Leonard J. Lyon, M.D.

Contents

Preface / v

1. **BASIC ELECTROCARDIOGRAPHY / 1**
   Basic Cardiac Anatomy and Physiology / 1
   The Electrocardiogram / 1
   Measuring Rates, Intervals and Axis from the
     Electrocardiogram / 9
   Technical Problems in Electrocardiography / 13

2. **CONDUCTION DISORDERS / 25**
   Normal Conduction Pathways / 25
   Atrioventricular Block / 26
   Intraventricular Block / 32
   Bifascicular and Trifascicular Block / 40

3. **DIAGNOSIS OF CARDIAC RHYTHMS / 44**
   Sinus Rhythms / 44
   Ectopic Rhythms / 45
   Premature Beats / 48
   Other Supraventricular Arrhythmias / 59
   Tachycardia-Bradycardia Syndrome / 80
   Ventricular Arrhythmias / 82

4. **MYOCARDIAL ISCHEMIA AND INFARCTION / 92**
   Acute Myocardial Infarction / 92
   Myocardial Ischemia / 94
   Location of Myocardial Infarction / 97
   Conduction Disorders in Myocardial Infarction / 109
   Arrhythmias in Acute Myocardial Infarction / 115

5. **ELECTROCARDIOGRAPHIC DIAGNOSIS IN OTHER DISEASES / 119**
    Acute Pericarditis / 119
    Pulmonary Embolism / 122
    Hyperkalemia / 126
    Hypokalemia / 131
    Preexcitation / 131

6. **DIGITALIS / 144**
    Digitalis Toxicity / 146
    Quiz / 148

7. **PACEMAKERS / 157**
    Principles and Uses / 157
    Recognizing Pacemaker Malfunction / 161
    Battery Depletion in Permanent Pacemakers / 165
    Pacemaker Follow-up / 165
    Correction of Malfunctions / 166

APPENDIX / 171

INDEX / 173

Basic Electrocardiography Handbook

CHAPTER 1
INTRODUCTION TO ELECTROCARDIOGRAPHY

BASIC CARDIAC ANATOMY AND PHYSIOLOGY

The heart is a muscular pump. The left side of the heart is the larger and thicker side. It does more work because it pumps oxygenated blood into the aorta (the main artery of the body) and then throughout the entire body. The thinner, right side of the heart pumps the same amount of blood, but only has to send it a short distance into the lungs via the pulmonary arteries. Each side of the heart consists of two chambers, an atrium and a ventricle. The thick-walled ventricles are the larger pumping chambers that expel blood from the heart with each beat (*contraction* or *systole*). The relatively thin-walled *atria* (older term: auricles) function as collecting and loading chambers. The atria hold blood being returned to the heart during ventricular systole. In between beats, the ventricles are relaxed (*diastole*). During diastole, blood flows into the ventricles from the atria—at first passively, and then propelled by atrial contraction (*atrial systole*). Strategically located valves prevent backflow of blood. The *mitral valve* is between the left atrium and ventricle, the *aortic valve* between the aorta and left ventricle, the *tricuspid valve* between the right ventricle and right atrium and the *pulmonary valve* between the main pulmonary artery and the right ventricle. These functions and relations are diagrammed in Figure 1-1.

THE ELECTROCARDIOGRAM

The electrocardiograph is a machine to record electrical currents picked up by special wires (*leads*, *electrodes*) attached to particular parts of the body. The heart is not the only source of recordable electric currents, however. Currents may be detected that originate in the muscles of the chest, the arms and the legs, from movements

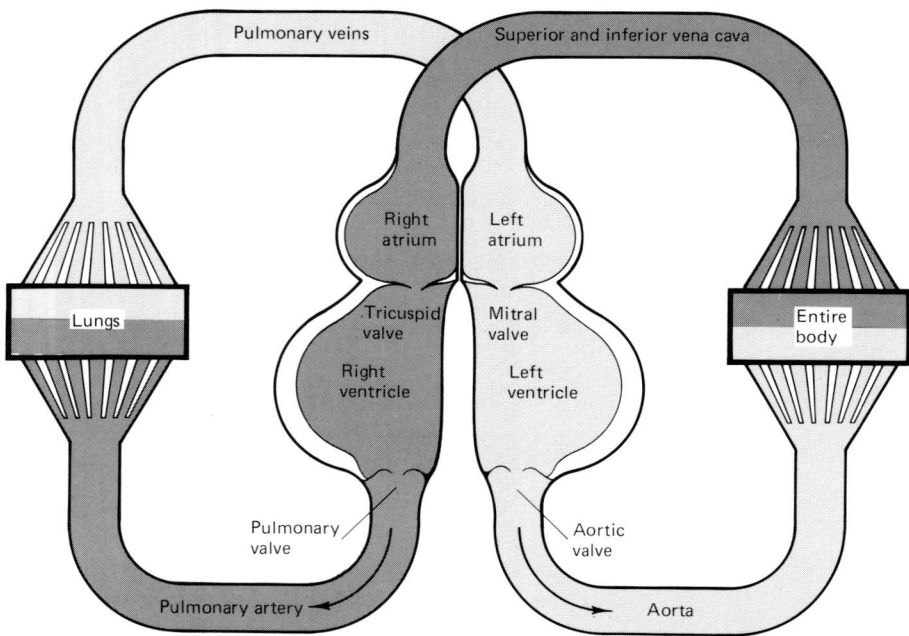

Figure 1-1.

of any part of the body, or even from sources outside the body such as electric beds or other electric equipment. The trick to taking a good *electrocardiogram* (recording made by an electrocardiograph machine) is to eliminate all the other sources of current so that the final record shows only electrical activity from the heart (see page 13, "Technical Problems").

When no current is flowing, the *stylus* (writing point) of the electrocardiograph does not move, and a straight line is recorded. A current flow causes a *deflection* (movement) of the stylus, so that a wave is inscribed on the ECG paper. Normal movements from the baseline are called *waves* and are designated P, QRS, T and U. The spaces between the waves which usually appear as straight lines are called *segments*, and are named by the waves they separate (for example, ST segment between the S and T waves). *Intervals* are also named by the waves at their beginning and end, for example, PR interval, but their measurement is from the beginning of the first wave, unlike the segments whose measurement starts at the end of the first wave. An interval ends with the start of the wave at its end just like a segment does, with one exception—the QT interval is measured from the start of the Q wave to the end of the T wave. The different waves, segments and intervals are diagrammed in Figure 1-2.

Each wave recorded on the electrocardiogram corresponds to a particular event in the cardiac cycle. Although the heart consists of several layers (Figure 1-3), it is only the heart muscle cell layer (myocardium) that generates currents large enough to be recorded by the electrocardiograph.

Figure 1-3 is a diagram of a cross section through the heart. The *endocardium* is a layer of smooth lining cells. These cells are found

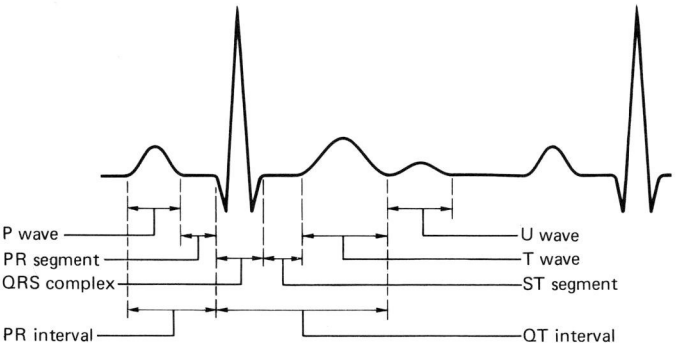

Figure 1-2.

not only in the heart, but also on the inside of all the blood vessels of the body, where they are called *endothelium*. The *myocardium* is the mass of heart muscle cells whose coordinated contraction causes the chambers of the heart to contract and pump blood. The myocardium is thin in the atria, thicker in the right ventricle and thickest in the left ventricle. The *epicardium* is a fatty layer on the outer surface of the myocardium. The major *coronary blood vessels*, the vessels that supply blood to the heart itself, run through the epicardium. The outermost layer is the *pericardium*, actually two layers with a small amount of lubricating fluid between them, forming the *pericardial sac* which encloses the entire heart.

Resting cardiac muscle cells (myocardial cells) maintain a small electrical charge across their cell membranes. Loss of this electrical charge (*depolarization*) occurs with a short, outward flow of current and initiates contraction of the muscle cells. After a short interval, the cells regain their charge (*repolarization*) with a short inward flow of current and are ready to contract again. The current recorded by the electrocardiograph at any moment is the sum of all the currents flowing in cells throughout the heart at that particular instant.

When current flows toward the recording electrode, the deflection is positive (upward), so that an upright wave will be recorded. Conversely, current flowing away from the electrode results in a negative (downward) deflection. If the current changes direction, as frequently happens, the result is a biphasic (up-and-down) wave. (See Figure 1-4.)

The first deflection of the cardiac cycle, the *P wave*, is caused by depolarization of the atria. The P wave is a small, rounded wave

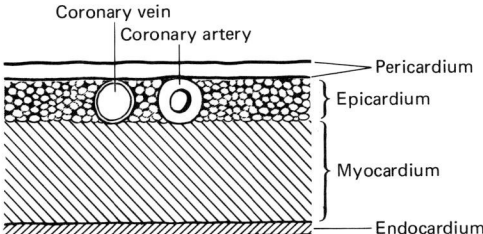

Figure 1-3.

4 / Basic Electrocardiography Handbook

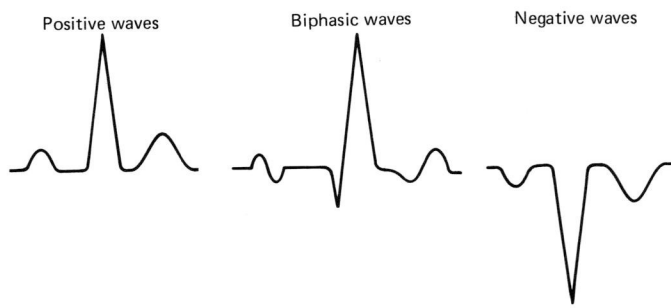

Figure 1-4. Wave forms.

which may be upright, notched, biphasic or inverted, depending on the particular lead being recorded. (See Figure 1-5.)

The *PR segment* (strictly speaking, the PQ segment, but conventionally referred to as the PR segment) separates the P from a large sharp deflection, the *QRS complex*, which is caused by depolarization of the ventricles. An atrial repolarization wave (*atrial T wave* or T_p wave) directed opposite to the P wave is seen occasionally, but usually is obscured by the QRS complex.

The QRS complex may consist of one sharp up-and-down wave, but more often it has several components, which are defined as follows (see Figure 1-6): The R wave is the first upward deflection; the Q wave is a downward deflection that precedes an R wave; the first downward deflection after the R wave is an S wave; if the entire complex is negative, it is called QS. There may be a second R wave—if so, it is designated R' (R prime); the second S wave is called S'; rarely, R" and S" are also present. To be separately labeled as part of the QRS, the wave must cross the baseline. Every wave changes direction once, but a second change which does not cross the baseline is called a notch.

An abrupt change in the direction of the wave marks the end of the QRS complex and the beginning of the ST segment. This point is called the J junction, or *J point*. The *ST segment* may be above ("elevated"), at or below ("depressed") the level of the baseline. The ST segment is followed by a large, rounded *T wave*, which corresponds to ventricular repolarization. The T wave may be notched, inverted or biphasic. Sometimes another rounded wave, the *U wave*, follows the T wave. The source of the U wave is uncertain. It is sometimes recorded from normal hearts, but when large it is often a sign of drug effect or electrolyte imbalance.

Although the chambers of the early embryonic heart are arranged like the diagram in Figure 1-1, by the time of birth the human heart has become folded on itself so that the chambers overlie one

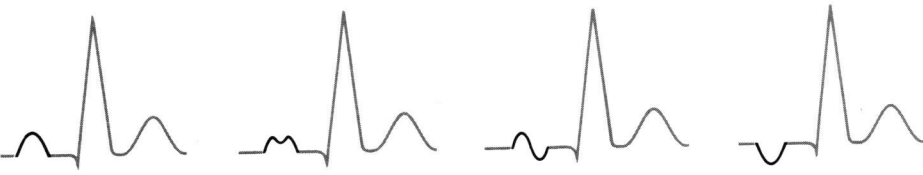

Figure 1-5. P waves.

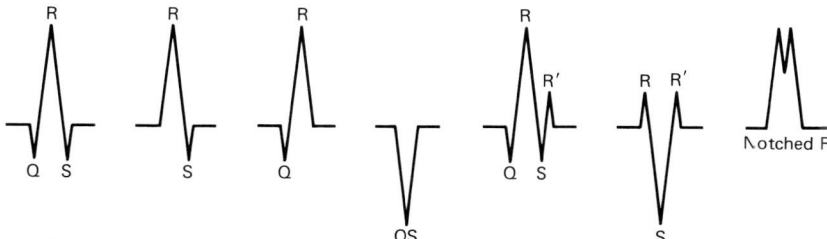

Figure 1-6. QRS complexes.

another. These spatial relationships are very important to visualize, because the electrocardiographic leads are placed around the heart in a specific arrangement. Since the electrocardiographic pattern recorded by each lead is largely determined by the parts of the heart the lead is facing, knowing the cardiac anatomy and its relationship to the ECG leads enables one to predict the normal pattern in each lead. Knowing the normal is a prerequisite to recognizing the abnormal.

Figure 1-7 shows a normal adult heart viewed from the front. Notice that the right ventricle is in front of (*anterior* to) the left ventricle as well as to its right. Similarly, the right atrium is anterior to, to the right of and somewhat below the left atrium. These relationships may also be appreciated in a horizontal slice made approximately at the level of the precordial (V) leads of the electrocardiogram (Figure 1-8).

Leads of the Electrocardiogram

The conventional electrocardiogram consists of 12 leads; that is, 12 different electrical views of the heart. The first six leads are the frontal plane leads. They include the three standard leads (I, II, III) and the three augmented limb leads (aV_R, aV_L and aV_F—usually

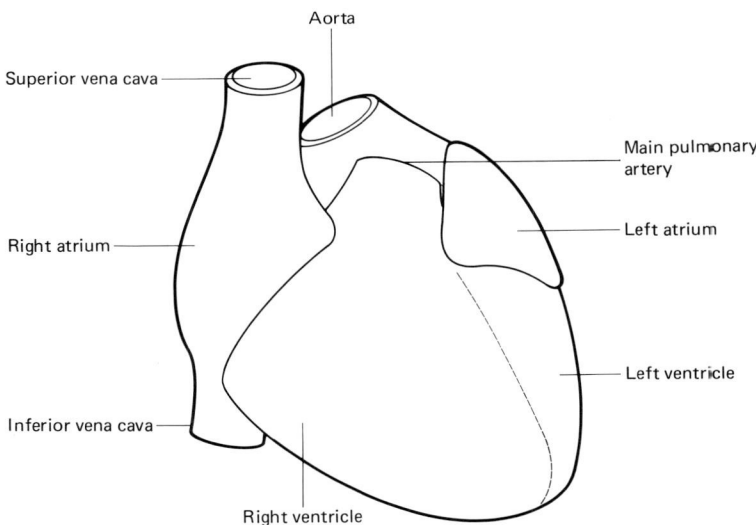

Figure 1-7.

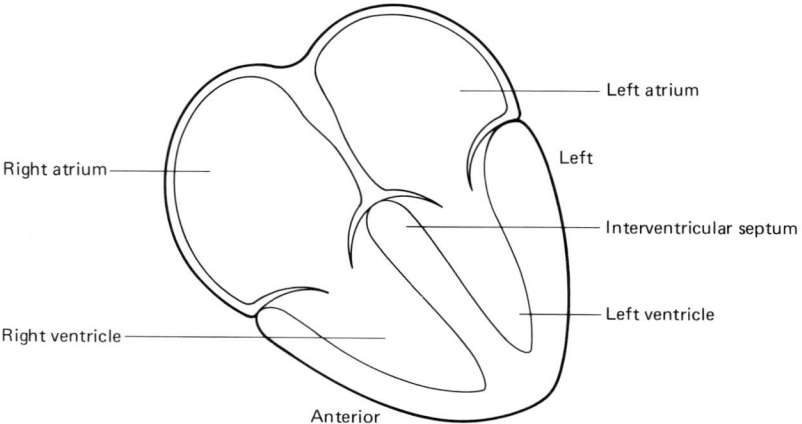

Figure 1-8.

referred to, for convenience, as R, L and F.* The name RoLF is a convenient mnemonic to help remember the sequence in which they are recorded). The electrocardiographic patterns recorded by the standard leads actually represent subtractions of the electrical potentials recorded by the limb leads. Thus,

$$I = L \text{ minus } R$$
$$II = F \text{ minus } R$$
$$III = F \text{ minus } L$$

These six leads look at the heart from the angles indicated in Figure 1-9, which also shows the average direction (*mean axis*) of atrial and ventricular depolarization (arrows leading from P and QRS, respectively). The largest positive deflections are always recorded by leads directly facing the mean axis of depolarization. Small, and frequently biphasic, complexes are recorded by leads perpendicular to the mean axis. Negative complexes appear in leads facing away from the mean axis (for example, lead R). Leads I, II, III, R, L and F register up and down and left and right forces, but not front and back.

The mean atrial electrical force, as recorded in the frontal plane leads, is directed leftward and inferiorly, because of the combined effects of left atrial depolarization (leftward) and right atrial depolarization (inferior); it is diagrammed in Figure 1-10. Therefore, the P wave is normally positive in leads I, II and F and negative in R. Either L or III or both should also record a positive P wave in a normal heart.

The earliest portion of the QRS complex reflects depolarization of the interventricular system, which proceeds from left to right (small arrow, Figure 1-9). Therefore, *a small initial negative wave ("septal" Q wave) is usually seen in leads I and L.* Since the left ventricular muscle mass is considerably greater than the right, left

---

*The letters correspond to *R*ight arm, *L*eft arm le*F*t leg electrodes. The right leg electrode is a ground.

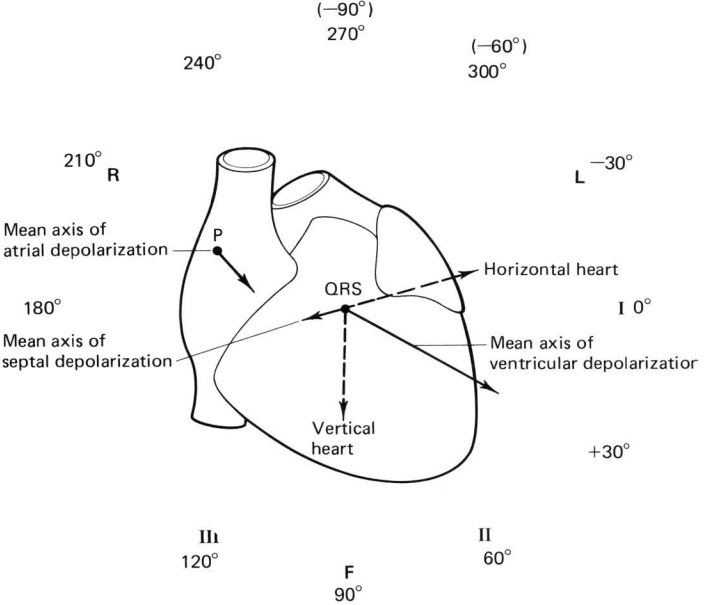

Figure 1-9. Frontal view of the heart showing the theoretical positions of leads I, II, III, R, L and F and the usual direction of atrial and ventricular depolarization.

ventricular forces dominate the remainder of the normal QRS complex, whose mean force is directed to the left and slightly inferiorly (large arrow). Therefore, *leads I and II should record a positive QRS*. Some variation of the electrical position of the heart may occur in normal persons of different physiques. For example, a more leftward placement ("*horizontal heart*") occurs in obese persons, who are, therefore, likely to have upright QRS complexes in leads I and L. In tall, slender individuals, the QRS is often shifted to the right. In such cases, predominantly negative complexes are recorded in L but positive ones in II, III and F ("*vertical heart*").

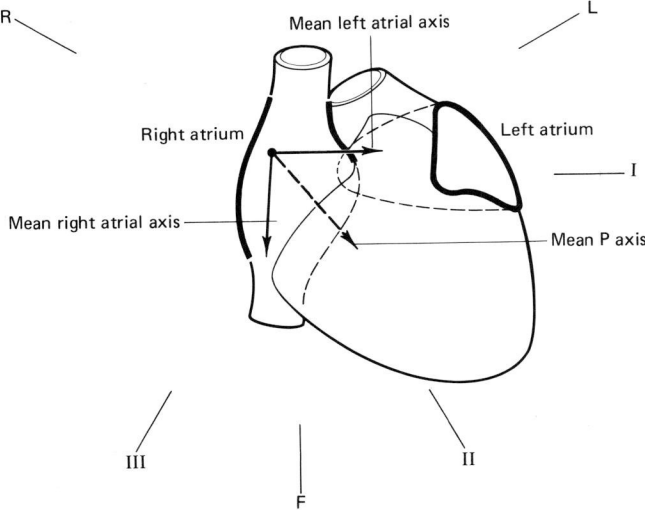

Figure 1-10.

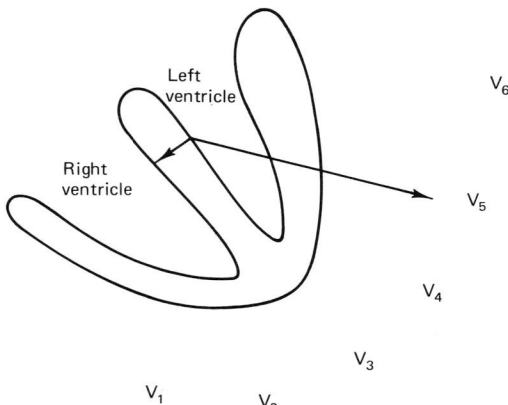

Figure 1-11.

T orientation is normally similar to that of the QRS complex. Therefore, in any lead, the predominant QRS and T deflections should go in the same direction, that is, both positive or both negative.

Figure 1-11 is a horizontal section through the heart, showing the approximate positions of the *precordial* (in front of the heart) *leads* (V_1-V_6). Each precordial lead records the myocardial electrical currents as seen from its point of view, and is most sensitive to changes in the myocardium nearest it. Therefore, leads V_1 and V_2 are most sensitive to events in the right side of the heart, and leads V_5 and V_6 to the left side. Sometimes, particularly in children, leads V_{3R} and V_{4R} (corresponding to V_3 and V_4 but on the right side of the chest) will be recorded to elicit possible evidence of right ventricular disease.

The earliest part of the QRS complex is caused by septal depolarization (smaller arrow, Figure 1-11). Because it goes from left to right, it causes a small positive deflection (R wave) in V_1 and a small negative deflection (septal Q wave) in V_6. The bulk of the QRS deflection reflects left ventricular depolarization. As a result most of the QRS complex is directed towards the left, resulting in a predominantly positive complex in V_5 and V_6 and a negative one in V_1.

Rhythm Strips and Monitor Leads

The conventional 12-lead electrocardiogram is intended to provide the interpreter with sufficient information to diagnose the cardiac rhythm and any disease involving one or more of the heart chambers. In some cases of abnormal heart rhythms (*arrhythmias*), the few beats shown in each lead are not enough for a definite diagnosis. This situation can be remedied by taking long recordings. Since the relationship between atrial and ventricular activity is often the key to diagnosing an arrhythmia, and since the QRS complexes are usually obvious in any lead, the rhythm strip should be made on a lead which best displays atrial activity. In most cases, this means lead II or V_1, but in all cases all 12 leads should be recorded first. The electrocardiograph operator can then select the best lead for a rhythm strip. If in doubt, one may take long strips of several leads and let the interpreter select.

Monitor leads are a special kind of rhythm strip. Cardiac *monitoring* (continuous observation) is used on patients who are likely to experience sudden changes in heart rhythm, and require immediate diagnosis and therapy should such changes occur. These situations include patients with acute myocardial infarction, patients undergoing general anesthesia, and patients with any condition serious enough to warrant intensive care. When cardiac monitoring is performed, a single lead is selected for continuous display on an oscilloscopic screen. Since the electrodes are attached to the patient's chest, the resulting complexes resemble those in a precordial lead. When the recording (positive) electrode is to the right of the sternum, the display is similar to V_1, which normally shows a negative QRS complex but is particularly useful for differentiating different types of bundle branch block (see Chapter 2 on "Conduction Disorders"). When the recording electrode is on the left chest, a V_5-like pattern results.

MEASURING RATES, INTERVALS AND AXIS FROM THE ELECTROCARDIOGRAM

Electrocardiographic paper is ruled in one-millimeter (mm) squares. Heavier lines are present every 5 mm. The vertical lines and, therefore, the number of boxes counted horizontally represent time. At the normal electrocardiographic paper speed of 25 mm per second, 25 little boxes equal one second, as do five large boxes. Each little box, therefore, is 1/25 or .04 second, and each large box is 1/5 or .2 second. Most electrocardiographic papers also include time markings in the margin, either every five large boxes (one second) or every 15 large boxes (3 seconds), indicated by the arrows in Figure 1-12.

The heart rate is the number of beats per minute. This may be calculated by counting the number of cycles (R-R or P-P intervals) in 6 seconds and multiplying by 10. Alternatively (and more cumbersomely), if the rhythm is regular, the rate may be calculated by dividing the number of little boxes in one cycle into 1,500. In some

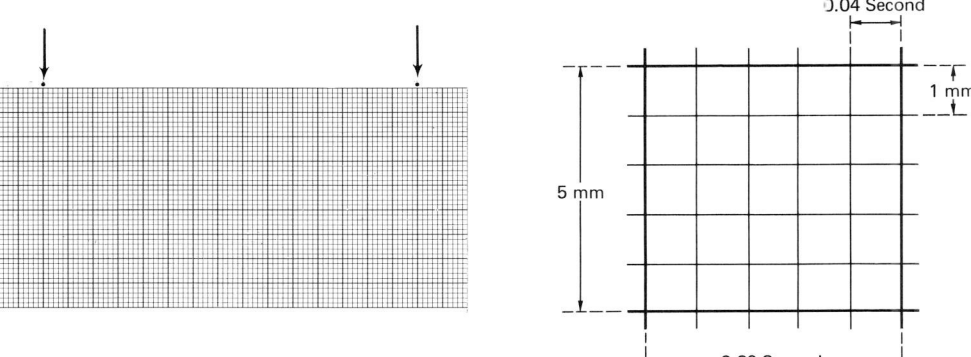

Figure 1-12.

cardiac arrhythmias, the atria and the ventricles do not beat at the same rate. In such cases, the atrial and ventricular rates should each be calculated.

The horizontal lines are for measurement of the electrical strength of various waves in millivolts. At the normal electrocardiographic *standardization* (setting), a one-millivolt deflection measures 10 millimeters (10 little boxes); so each little box is 0.1 millivolt going up or down. When disease causes a heart chamber to enlarge, one of the best electrocardiographic signs is an increase in the height of the wave generated by that chamber—for example, in left ventricular *hypertrophy* (muscular thickening) the R wave is abnormally tall in leads V_5 and V_6.

Figure 1-13 is a lead II rhythm strip from a healthy patient to illustrate how these measurements are made. In 30 large boxes counted horizontally (6 seconds) there are 8¼ cycles; so the heart rate is 10 × 8¼ or about 82 beats per minute. The R waves are not exactly the same height (they vary as the heart moves in the chest while the patient breathes), but all are between eight and nine little boxes tall; so the R wave is .8 to .9 millivolt.

Four other important electrocardiographic measurements are the PR interval, the QRS duration, the QT interval and the frontal QRS axis. The *PR interval* extends from the beginning of the P wave to the beginning of the QRS complex. The normal PR interval may be as short as .12 second (three little boxes) or as long as .20 second (five little boxes). The *QRS duration* is measured from the beginning to the end of the QRS complex; it is the time required for the ventricles to become completely depolarized, and should not exceed .10 second. The PR interval and the QRS duration are two particularly important measurements for evaluating conduction within the heart.

The *QT interval* extends from the beginning of the QRS complex to the end of the T wave. The QT interval varies with the heart rate, shortening in duration as the heart rate increases. Tables are available listing the normal QT interval for any given heart rate.

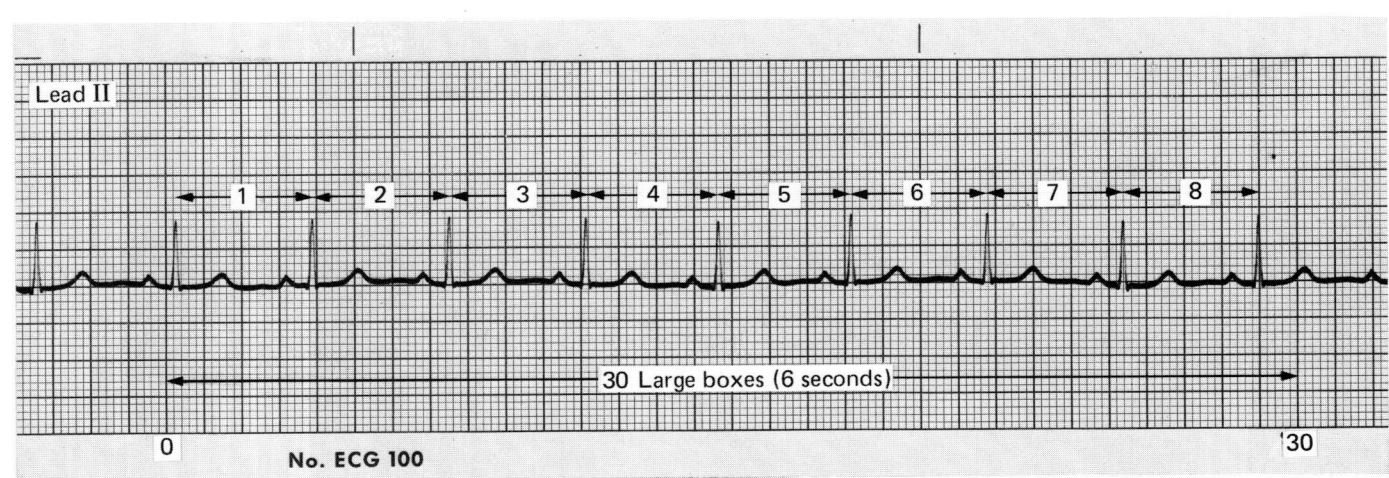

Figure 1-13.

As a rule of thumb, however, for a normal heart rate (60–100 beats per minute) the QT should be less than .40 second. When the QT interval is prolonged, the heart is at greater risk of developing serious and potentially fatal arrhythmias.

The *mean frontal QRS axis* is a measurement of the direction of the average QRS force in the frontal plane, the plane which contains the first six electrocardiographic leads (I, II, III, R, L, F). Normally, the mean frontal QRS axis falls between −30° and +90°. There are methods for precise computation of the QRS axis, but what is really important is to know whether the axis is normal, or abnormally shifted to the left (*abnormal left axis deviation*) or right (*abnormal right axis deviation*) (Figure 1-14). This may be determined in most cases merely by inspecting leads I and II.

Since +90° is perpendicular to lead I, then if the positive forces of the QRS (R wave) exceed the negative forces (Q plus S waves) in lead I, the axis is to the left of +90°. In other words, abnormal right axis deviation is not present. Because the electrocardiogram looks at the heart from the front, "left" means the patient's left, not the observer's. On the other hand, if the negative forces predominate in lead I, abnormal right axis deviation is present. The same process is applied to lead II to determine if abnormal left axis deviation is present. If R is larger than Q plus S in II, then abnormal left axis deviation is not present. On the other hand, if R in II is smaller than Q plus S, abnormal left axis deviation is present. This method fails in only two circumstances, both of which are uncommon: (1) when the axis deviation is so abnormal that the mean frontal axis falls between −90° and +150°, you might conclude that it is both abnormal right and abnormal left axis deviation, but this is impossible since only one can be present at a time; (2) when RS or QR patterns are present in many leads with the positive and

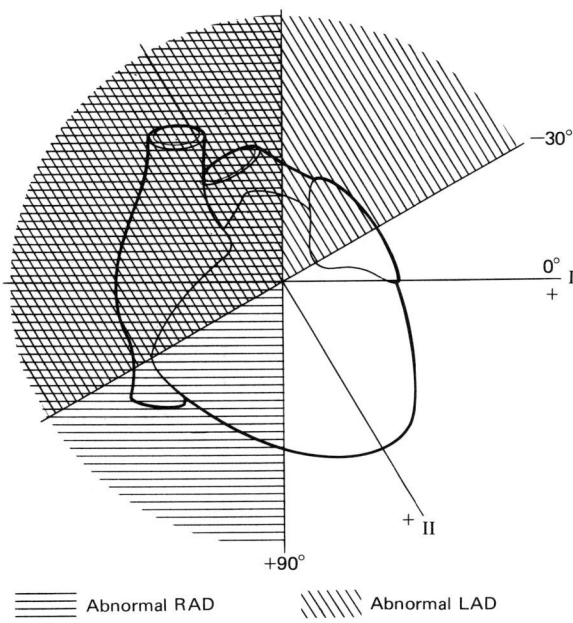

Figure 1-14.

12 / Basic Electrocardiography Handbook

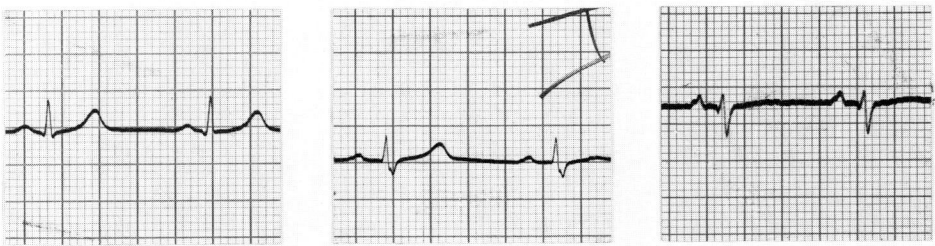

Figure 1-15.

negative waves approximately equal in size, the axis is *indeterminate* by either this or any other method.

Figure 1-15 shows some QRS complexes recorded in lead I to

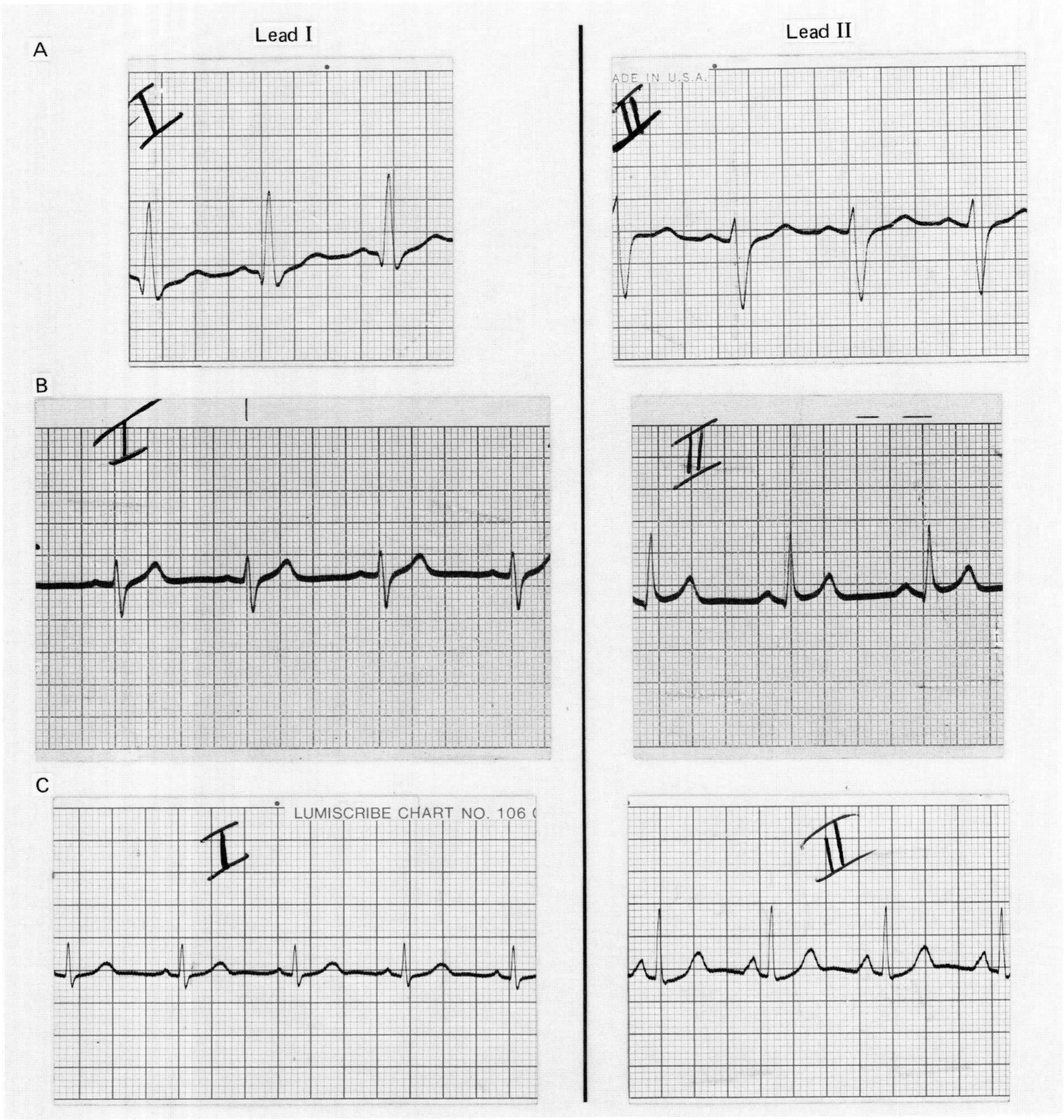

Figure 1-16.

NO POSTAGE
NECESSARY
IF MAILED
IN THE
UNITED STATES

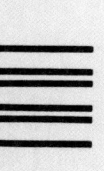

BUSINESS REPLY CARD
FIRST CLASS   Permit No. 1   Pleasantville, N.Y.

POSTAGE WILL BE PAID BY ADDRESSEE

**Reader's Digest
Pleasantville
New York 10570**

ORDER CERTIFICATE

FILL OUT, DETACH, AND MAIL TODAY!

23038

1 0047 11513 08531 X   02815
MR L. HORNICK
3 KNIGHTS HILL CT.
HUNTINGTON STA, NY 11746

22848

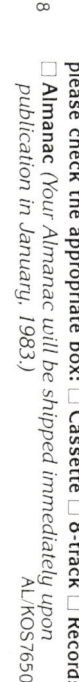

YES! Please send me for 7 days home-trial the Reader's Digest product(s) of my choice, indicated below. You will bill me the low price listed (plus postage, and applicable state tax, if any), with no charge for handling. (Price and postage subject to change without notice.) If I am not satisfied, I may return the product(s), owe nothing, and you will reimburse me for the postage. Order subject to acceptance and credit approval by Reader's Digest.

To order Kings of Swing
please check the appropriate box: ☐ **Cassette** ☐ **8-track** ☐ **Records**

☐ **Almanac** *(Your Almanac will be shipped immediately upon publication in January, 1983.)*

AL/KOS7650

illustrate application of this method of axis deviation determination. In the case on the left, the R wave is much larger than the Q wave plus the S wave; so right axis deviation is not present. In the middle example, the R and S waves are about equal in area. This indicates borderline right axis deviation. In the right-hand case, Q plus S are much larger than R, so abnormal right axis deviation is present.

Review Cases

Figure 1-16 shows leads I and II recorded from three different patients. Measure the heart rate, PR interval, QRS duration and QT interval in each case. Note whether the QT interval is prolonged, and check for abnormal axis deviation.

Answers: Case A. The heart rate has to be determined by dividing the RR interval (18 small boxes) into 1,500 since the strips are not long enough to count the number of cycles in 6 seconds. Fifteen hundred divided by 18 is 83.333; but since we always round off the heart rate to the nearest whole number, the answer is 83 beats per minute. The PR interval is .18 second (4½ small boxes). The QRS duration is .16 second (four small boxes). The QT interval is .44 second (11 small boxes)—since it is longer than .40 second, it is prolonged. In lead I the R wave is larger than Q plus S, so there is no abnormal right axis deviation; but in II, S is much larger than R, so abnormal left axis deviation is present.

Case B. The heart rate is 75 if you measured it in lead I, 71 in lead II. The heart rate often changes slightly during the electrocardiogram; so select any representative area for your calculations. The PR interval is .16 second. If you said .17 second, that's close enough. I hope you measured in lead II—the P wave is larger there, and it is easier to see where it starts. The QT interval is .34 second (normal). S larger than R in lead I indicates abnormal right axis deviation.

Case C. The heart rate is 88 beats per minute (1,500 divided by 17). The PR interval is .15 second, but if you said .14 or .16, that's acceptable. The QT interval is .34 second (normal). R is larger than S in leads I and II; so there is no abnormal axis deviation.

TECHNICAL PROBLEMS IN ELECTROCARDIOGRAPHY

There is more to taking an electrocardiogram than merely attaching the leads to the patient and turning on the machine. There are many details that must be attended to so that the final result is an electrocardiogram of high enough quality to enable the reader to identify even subtle electrocardiographic abnormalities.

Most electrocardiograph manufacturers provide instruction booklets that review the different controls on the machine and the possible sources of error in recording an electrocardiogram. You should familiarize yourself with your machine's instructional manual before you start recording electrocardiograms.

Errors in recording electrocardiograms produce various kinds of distortions in the record. In many cases, these distortions make the electrocardiogram difficult or impossible to interpret; thus the electrocardiogram has to be repeated or—even worse—if the condition requiring the electrocardiogram is no longer present, the chance for making a diagnosis has been lost. These errors are recognizable while the tracing is being taken; therefore as soon as you see one of them, you should stop and make the necessary correction and then take a good electrocardiogram. This section will illustrate some of the common errors and how they can be corrected.

Correct and Incorrect Standardization

After the leads have been attached to the patient and the machine turned on long enough to allow it to warm up—usually about a minute—the machine should be standardized. The instruction manual will tell you how to do this on your particular machine, but the essence of the procedure is the recording of a measured one-millivolt signal. When the machine is correctly set, this test signal will cause a deflection of exactly 10 mm (10 little boxes). If the deflection is not exactly 10 little boxes as measured from the top of the baseline to the top of the calibration signal, the appropriate adjustment must be made before the electrocardiogram is taken.

Whenever possible, an electrocardiogram should be recorded at normal standardization. Occasionally, in some leads the QRS complex is so large that it will not fit on the paper unless the recording is made at half standardization (one millivolt equals 5 mm). When this change is made, it must be clearly indicated on the recording paper, so that anyone interpreting the electrocardiogram will realize what has been done.

Sometimes, usually by error resulting from failure to inspect the standardization, an entire electrocardiogram is recorded at half standard (Figure 1-17). This results in abnormally small QRS complexes and P and T waves that are difficult to interpret because of their small size, and might suggest a number of serious diseases that cause truly low-voltage electrocardiograms unless the interpreter happens to notice the standardization.

Although it is not done as often as recording at half standardization, it is also possible to record an electrocardiogram at double standardization (one millivolt equals 20 mm). The purpose of recording at double standardization is to magnify the electrical signals so that small waves can be seen more easily. When an electrocardiogram is mistakenly recorded at double standard, all the waves come out twice as large as they should, and unless the error is detected by the reader, the electrocardiogram may be interpreted as showing atrial and ventricular hypertrophy.

Incorrect Paper Speed

Normal recording speed is 25 mm per second, meaning that 25 mm of paper passes the stylus each second. Most electrocardiographs have a switch that permits advancing the paper at double

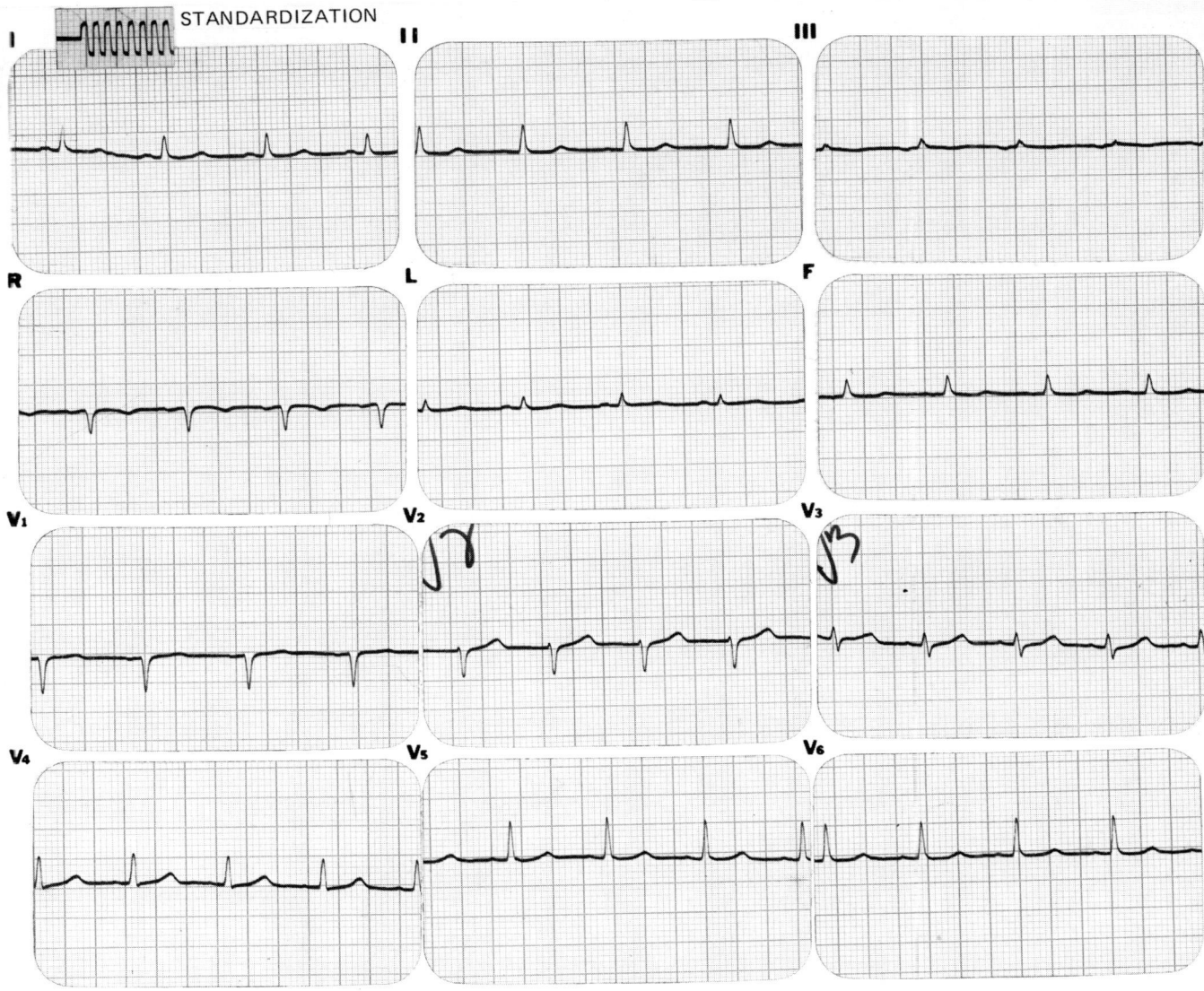

Figure 1-17.

speed (50 mm per second). If an electrocardiogram is mistakenly taken at this setting, the result looks like a patient with an abnormally slow heart rate, abnormally wide QRS complexes and abnormally long PR and QT intervals. These "abnormalities" can be seen in Figure 1-18, which was recorded at double speed from the same healthy person whose half-standardized electrocardiogram was shown in Figure 1-17. Since Figure 1-18 was correctly standardized, the QRS complexes do appear at their normal height—twice what they seemed to be in Figure 1-17.

Lead Reversal

Although the electrocardiographic leads are clearly labeled ("right arm," "right leg," etc.) and usually color-coded as well, from time to time they manage to get attached to the wrong limb anyway.

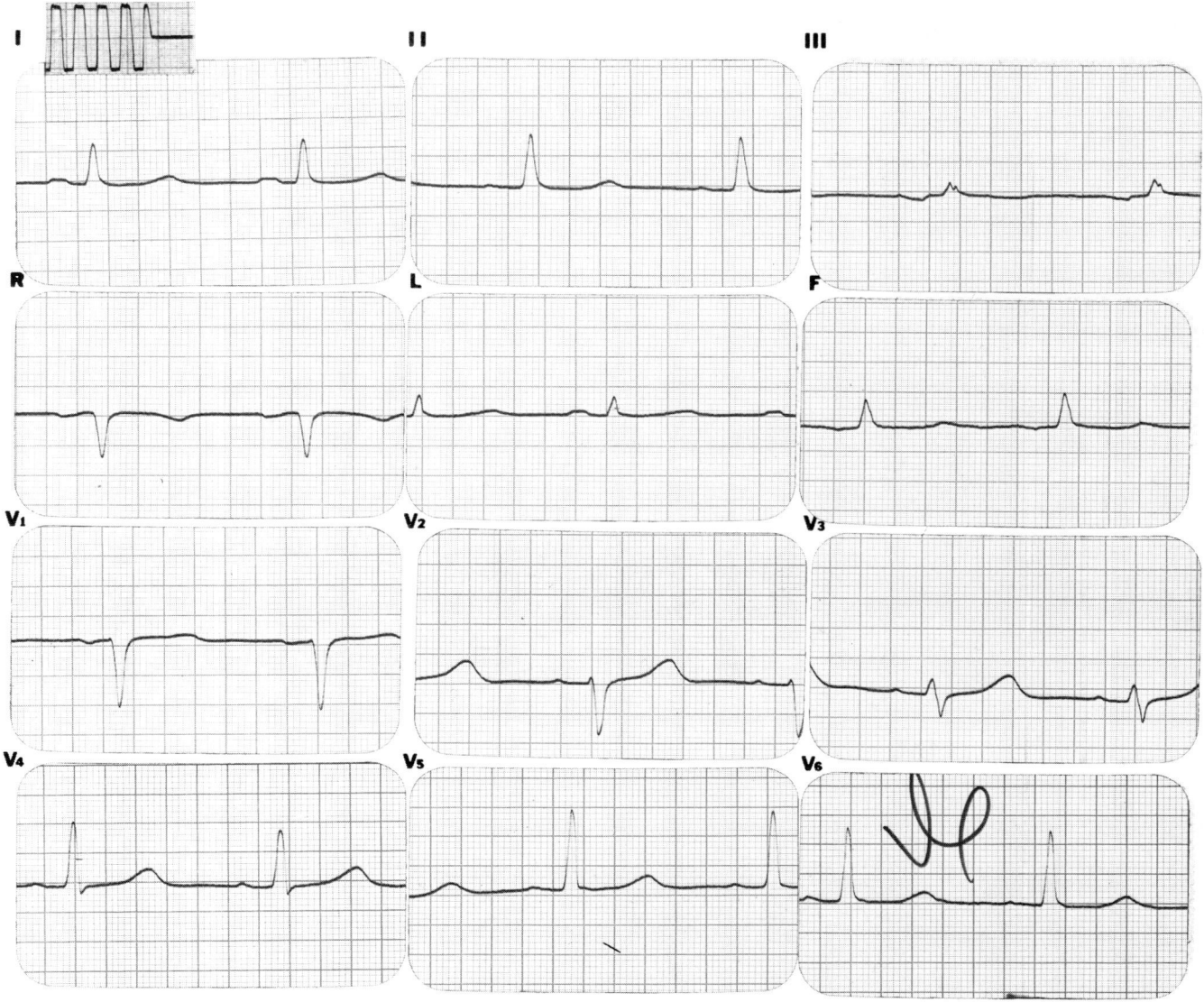

Figure 1-18.

The laws of mathematics indicate that there are 24 different possible arrangements of four electrodes on four limbs, and 120 if you manage to mix up the V lead cable with one of the limb leads. Yet, despite this multitude of possibilities, the most common error is reversal of the arm electrodes so that the right arm lead is attached to the left arm and vice versa. Since lead I is the difference in potential between the two arms (left minus right), with the arm leads reversed, lead I will now show right minus left, so that the recording of lead I will be the normal lead I upside down. Figure 1-19 is such a case. Incidentally, notice the perfect standardization in the middle of lead I, the mark of an experienced technician. However, the P, QRS and T waves are still inverted. Although these inversions can be seen in dextrocardia, a rare congenital condition where the heart is turned around in the chest, at least 95% of the time they are caused by reversal of the limb electrodes. So if you see that everything is

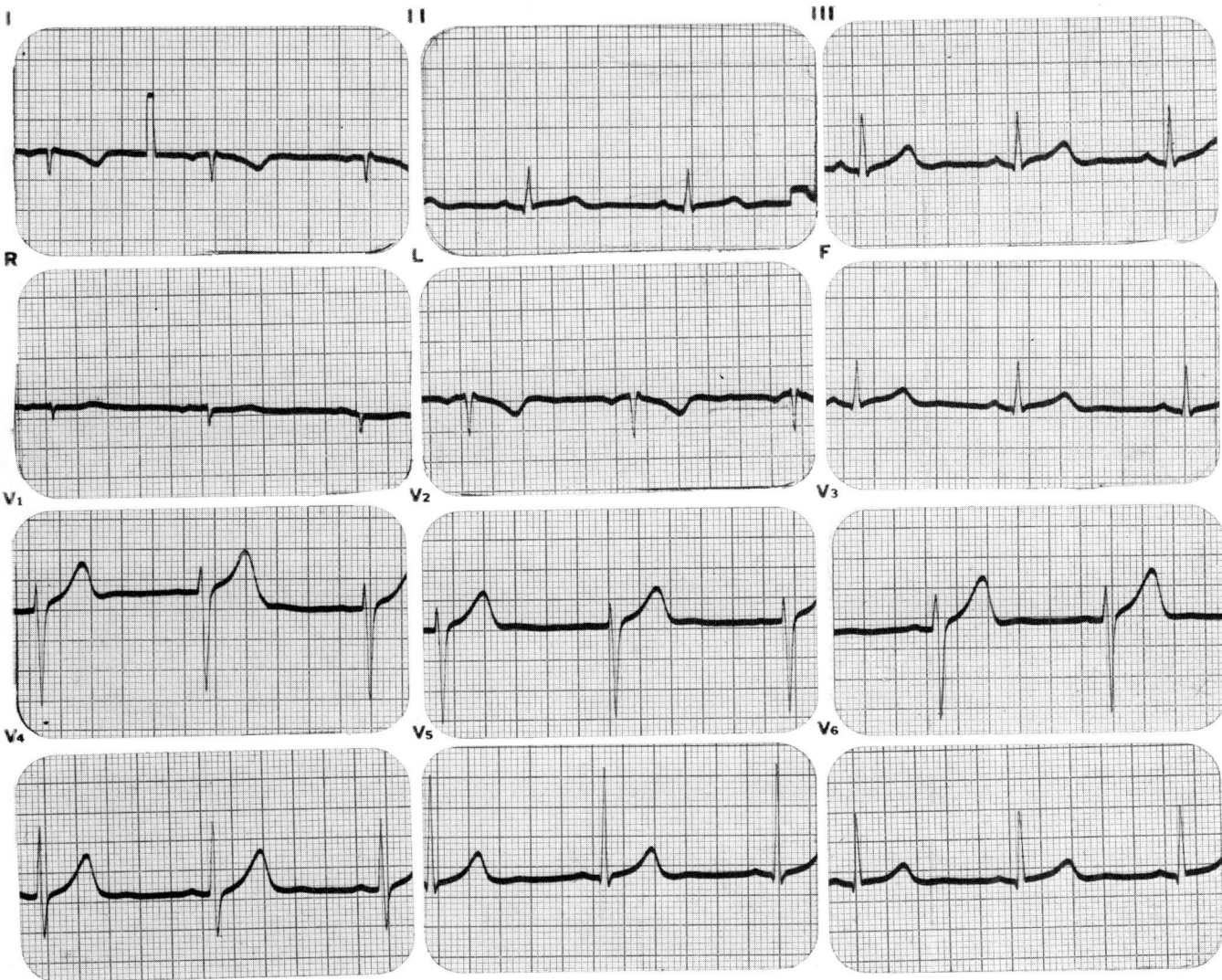

Figure 1-19.

inverted in lead I, check the limb electrodes before taking the rest of the electrocardiogram.

Imprecise Placement of Precordial Electrodes

Placement of the precordial electrodes is not as easy as placing the limb electrodes, because the suction cup or equivalent device at the end of the V lead cable must be put on precise locations across the chest. Correct placement of the V leads depends on locating certain anatomic landmarks: the sternal angle, the fourth and fifth intercostal spaces and the midclavicular, anterior and midaxillary lines. The task becomes even more difficult in hairy-chested men, large-breasted women and patients who already have wires on, bandages on or tubes in their chests. All too many people are careless about this aspect of electrocardiographic recording. However, the result of imprecise precordial electrode placement is that it becomes impossible to evaluate day-to-day changes in the V leads, so that potentially important diagnostic information is lost. In summary, take your time and be accurate in placing the precordial leads.

Smeared Electrode Paste

Another common error in recording precordial leads is excessive use of electrode paste. The purpose of electrode paste is to lower the electrical resistance of the skin so that the heart's currents can be recorded. Use only enough to cover the area where the electrode will be applied, because the electrode will record from the entire area covered with paste. If the operator applies so much paste that the glob for V_2 touches that for V_3, and that one is in contact with the paste for V_4 and so on to V_6, the result is that leads V_{2-6} will all come out looking pretty much alike.

Respiratory Motion

The heart changes its position within the chest each time a person breathes in or out. If the patient is comfortable and relaxed while the electrocardiogram is being recorded, the movements of the heart will be too slight to affect the cardiogram. However, if the patient is breathing deeply and rapidly because of either anxiety or a disease causing true shortness of breath, then the respiratory movements of the heart may cause a major distortion. Respiratory movements, which may be seen in any lead but as a rule are most prominent in the precordial leads, cause a cyclical rising and falling of the baseline, corresponding to the phases of respiration (Figure 1-20). The only way to eliminate respiratory motion artefact is to make the patient as comfortable as possible, be reassuring, and, in some cases, ask the patient to stop breathing. Even very sick patients can usually hold their breath for 3 to 4 seconds, which is all the time you need to obtain a good recording of one lead. When you ask the patient to stop breathing, make sure it is done without his first taking a very deep breath, because a full inspiration will alter the heart's usual position and may cause certain reflexes that drastically slow the heart rate. And, of course, when you have obtained 3 to 4 seconds of good recording, be sure to tell the patient to breathe again.

60 Cycle Artefact

In this country, electricity is delivered to users as 60 cycle alternating current. This means that the direction of flow of electricity in all electric wires changes 60 times a second. When either the patient or the electrocardiograph is improperly grounded so that outside current is detected, the result is a distortion of the electrocardiogram by 60 sharp up-and-down waves a second, so-called 60 cycle artefact as shown in Figure 1-21.

No one can interpret an electrocardiogram with 60 cycle artefact, so the cause of the artefact must be found and corrected. Some

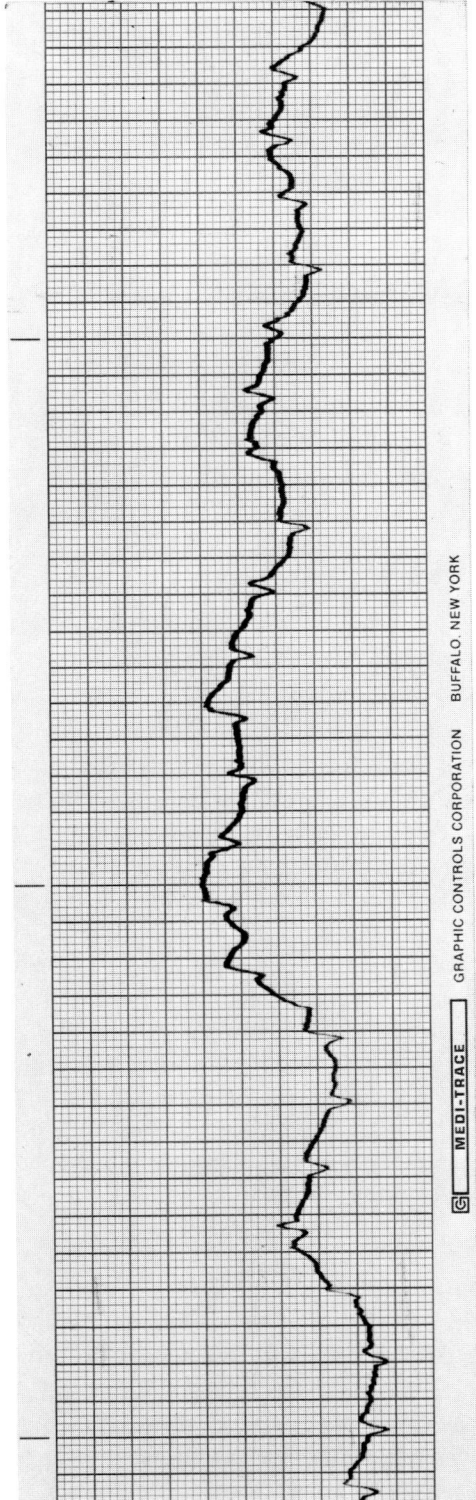

Figure 1-20.

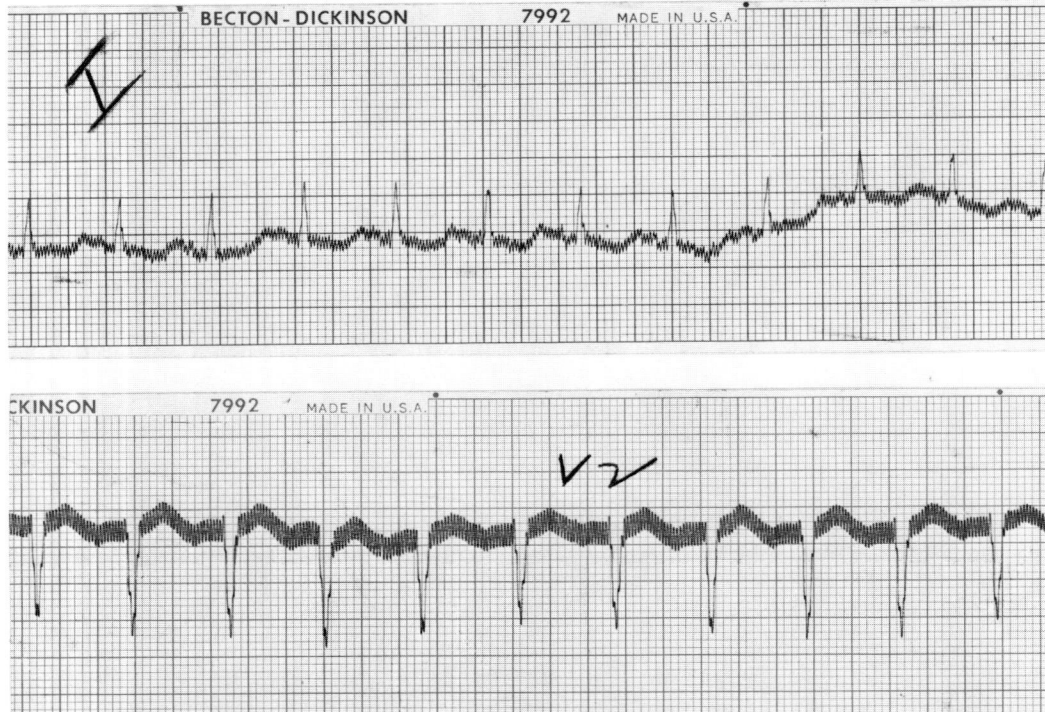

Figure 1-21.

common causes and their cures are: (1) the patient's hand or foot touching the metal bedframe, even of a nonelectric bed—move the hand or foot; (2) one of the limb leads not connected to the patient—make sure all leads are firmly fastened; (3) 60 cycle artefact in the precordial leads only, which usually means a disconnected V lead; (4) an improperly grounded electric bed—unplug the bed while taking the electrocardiogram. In past years, improper grounding of the electrocardiograph was a common cause of 60 cycle artefact. However, with hospitals wired according to current standards and modern electrocardiographs with grounded (three-way) plugs, 60 cycle artefact due to improper grounding should rarely be a problem.

Artefact from Loose Electrodes

If an electrode is loosely attached to a patient, the recording plate or suction cup can rock back and forth on the patient's skin. Every such movement causes a wavy deflection of the baseline resembling that caused by atrial fibrillation (Chapter 3). However, in almost all cases of atrial fibrillation, the RR intervals are completely irregular. Therefore, if the baseline is wavy but the RR intervals are regular, look for a loose electrode. Figure 1-22 is a three-channel electrocardiogram in which V_1, V_2 and V_3 were recorded simultaneously. The wavy baseline in V_1 looks just like atrial fibrillation. However, simultaneous recordings from V_2 and V_3 show a perfectly normal rhythm with a P wave preceding each QRS complex, proving that the "atrial fibrillation" in lead V_1 was really a loose-electrode

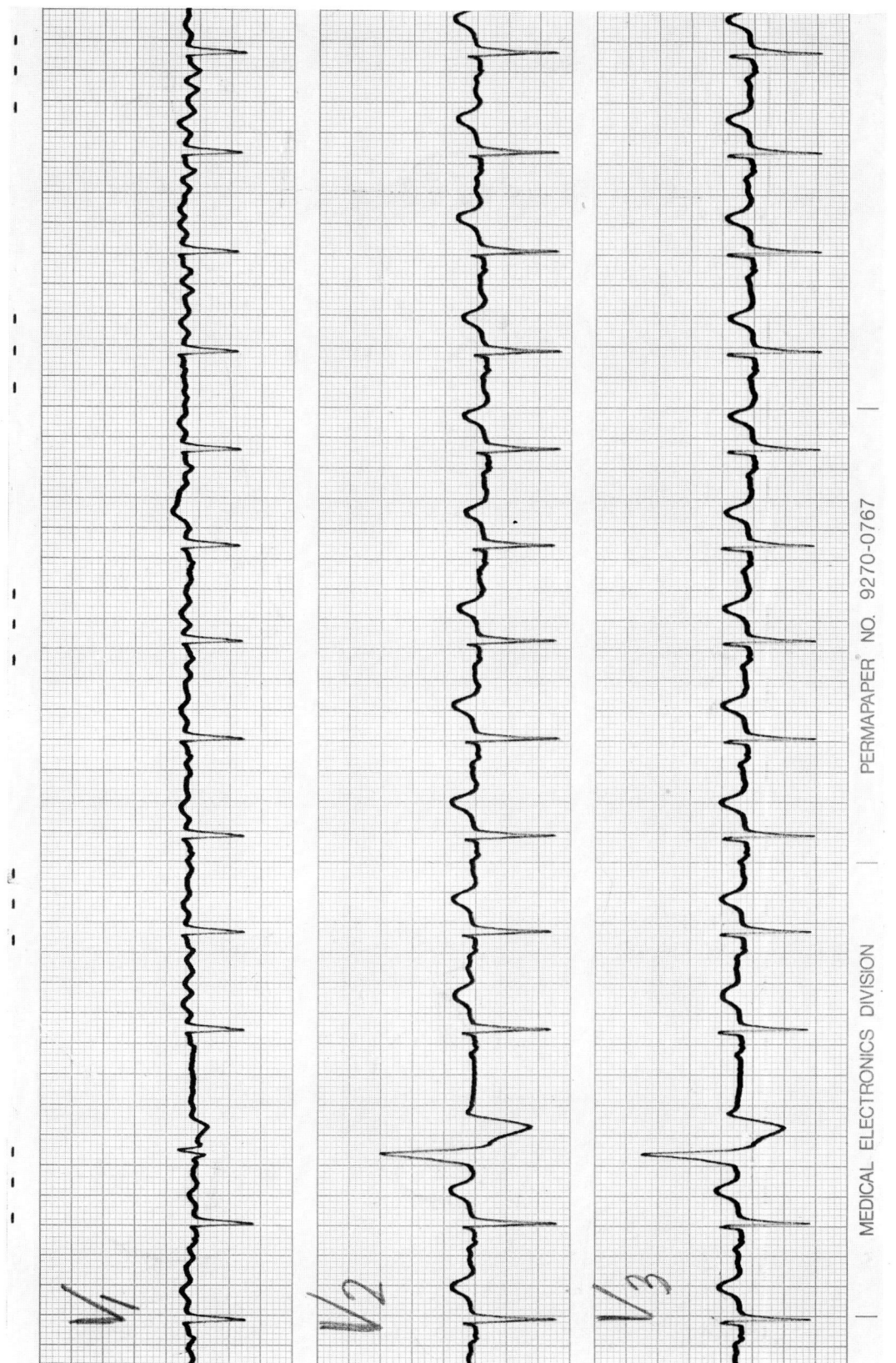

Figure 1-22.

22 / Basic Electrocardiography Handbook

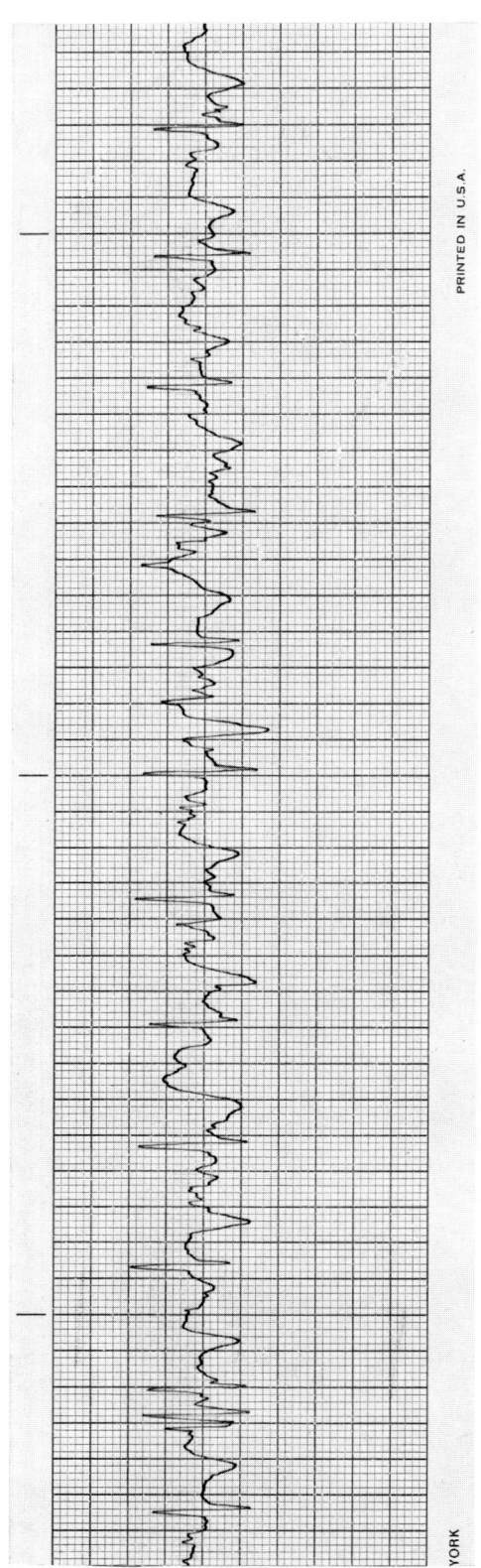

Figure 1-23.

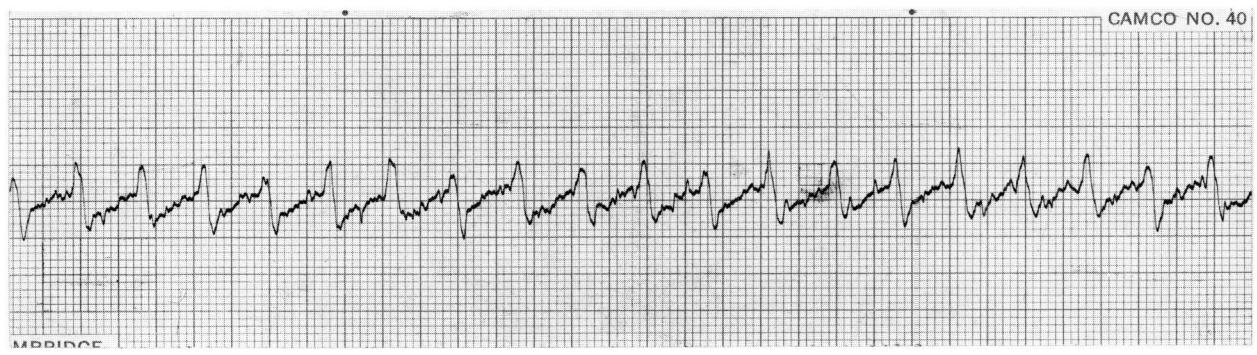

Figure 1-24.

artefact. The artefact was eliminated by securely reapplying the electrode.

Occasionally, loose-electrode artefact takes the form of sharp up-and-down deflections that may occur singly or in bunches. This situation is illustrated by Figure 1-23, a rhythm strip recorded from a cardiac monitor. Again, the regular RR interval is a clue that this is probably not a true electrocardiogram.

Artefact from Skeletal Muscle Tremor

Movement of an arm or a leg during the recording of an electrocardiogram causes a baseline deflection; so patients are always told to lie still during the test. However, even while lying still, a person who is very cold or very tense or very uncomfortable will be contracting many of his body's muscles. Muscle artefact looks something like the artefact of a loose electrode, except that the waves are usually sharper like those shown in Figure 1-24. To eliminate tremor artefact, make sure the patient is comfortable. If he is cold, a blanket may help. If he is holding his arms stiffly, ask him to place his hands under his buttocks. Check for excessive tension on the electrode cables, because if they are pulled tight, they will magnify skeletal muscle currents. Finally, make sure that there is a good contact between the electrode terminal and the skin—this is best achieved by rubbing the electrode paste into the skin with the terminal plate or suction cup.

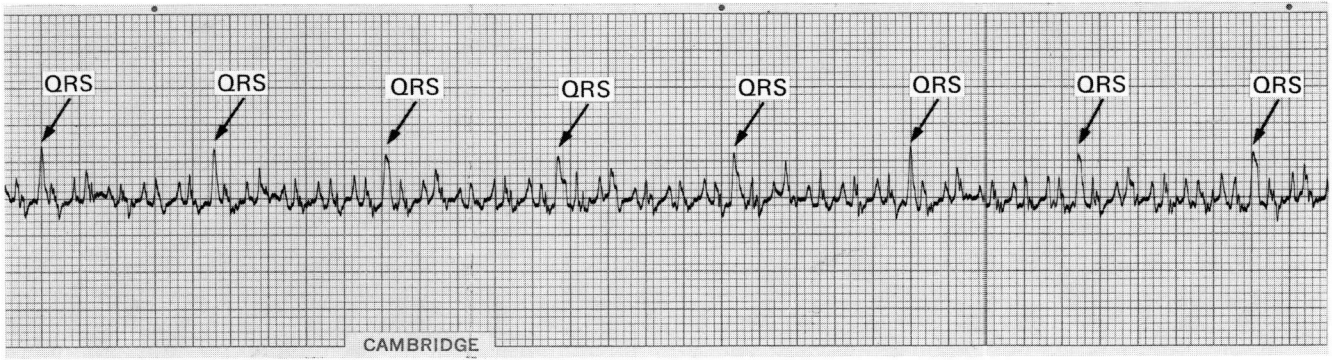

Figure 1-25.

Table 1-1. Electrocardiographic Findings That Suggest Recording Errors

Finding	Possible source of error
Low voltage complexes	Recording at ½ standardization
High voltage complexes	Recording at double standardization
Wide QRS complexes and slow heart rate	Recording at double speed
All waves inverted in I	Reversed arm electrodes
V leads change from day to day without corresponding changes in I or L	Imprecise V lead placement
Many V leads look the same	Smearing of electrode paste
Baseline moves up and down	Respiratory motion
60 cycle artefact	Patient touching bed frame / Disconnected electrode / Improperly grounded electric bed
Wavy baseline with regular RR intervals / Sharp, irregular baseline deflections	Loose electrode / Skeletal muscle tremor

In some cases, rapid, rhythmic muscle tremor artefacts will be recorded from patients with certain neurologic disorders such as Parkinson's Disease. Figure 1-25 is an extreme example where the muscle tremor artefacts caused by the Parkinsonian tremor almost hide the QRS complexes. Unfortunately, in such a case nothing you can do will completely eliminate the tremor. Nevertheless, most patients with tremor from neurologic disease will shake more when they are anxious and less when they are relaxed; so the more you reassure the patient and allay his anxieties, the better your electrocardiogram will turn out.

Table 1-1 summarizes the common errors in electrocardiogram recording, and the clues that should help you diagnose what you are doing wrong.

Chapter 2
Conduction Disorders

NORMAL CONDUCTION PATHWAYS

For the heart to pump blood effectively, the myocardial cells of each chamber must contract in a coordinated way. This coordination is achieved by electrical signals (*impulses*) which originate in the *sinoatrial (SA) node*, the heart's own pacemaker. These impulses are conducted over specialized tissues to reach all parts of the heart at the proper time. The impulses are strong enough to stimulate first the atria then the ventricles to to contract, but are too weak to be detected on the ordinary electrocardiogram. Nevertheless, malfunctions of any part of the conducting system can be readily diagnosed, since they cause delayed depolarization of the atria, the ventricles, one ventricle or even part of one ventricle, resulting in characteristic changes in the electrocardiographic pattern.

Figure 2-1 shows the most important structures in the heart's electrical system. The sinoatrial node is located in the right atrium near the point of entrance of the superior vena cava. The sinoatrial node emits 70 to 80 electrical impulses per minute (or more, or less, according to the body's needs). These impulses then spread through the atrial myocardium (light dashed lines, Figure 2-1), causing the atria to contract and giving rise to P waves on the electrocardiogram.

At the same time that a sinoatrial impulse spreads throughout the atria, it also travels over special bundles of atrial tissue to the *atrioventricular (AV) node*, located where the walls of the atria and ventricles meet (the *AV junction*). (This path is indicated by the heavy dashed lines in Figure 2-1.) The impulse is then conducted slowly through the AV node. Delay of the impulse in the AV node allows enough time for atrial systole to complete the process of ventricular filling. This delay also accounts for most of the PR interval on the electrocardiogram.

Once the impulse leaves the lower AV node, it travels very rapidly

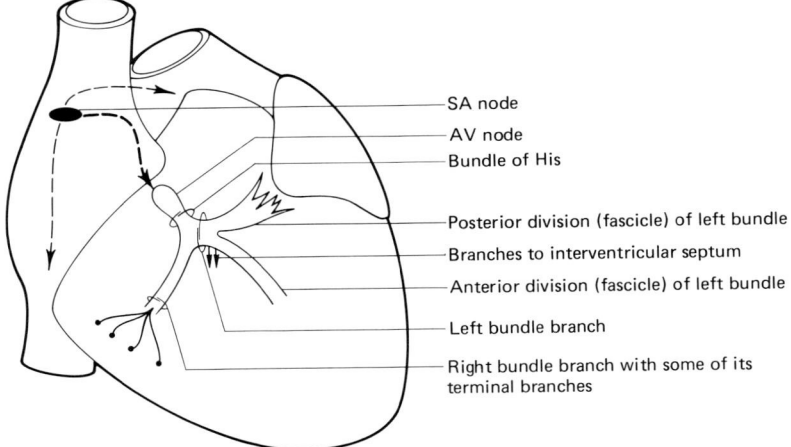

Figure 2-1.

over myocardial cells specialized for electrical conduction, the *Purkinje cells*. These cells are organized into a cable-like structure, the *Bundle of His*. The Bundle of His soon divides. The long, slender *right bundle branch* carries the impulse to its terminal branches, which distribute it to the right ventricular myocardium. The *left bundle branch* is much thicker and shorter than the right bundle branch. After giving off a few short branches to the interventricular septum, the left bundle branch divides into a thin *left anterior division (fascicle)* and a thicker *left posterior division (fascicle)*. Each of these fascicles eventually divides and delivers the impulse to the left ventricular myocardium via a network of terminal branches similar to those in the right ventricle.

ATRIOVENTRICULAR BLOCKS

Any abnormality of impulse conduction between the atria and ventricles is called *atrioventricular (AV) block*. This includes abnormally slow conduction and the failure of some or all atrial impulses to reach the ventricles. Accurate diagnosis of AV block permits a reasonable estimate of the location of the block (Figure 2-2), and this in turn indicates the seriousness of the condition and the likelihood that pacemaker therapy (Chapter 7) will be required. AV block is divided into the following categories:

1. First degree AV block
2. Second degree AV block
    Type I
    Type II
    2:1 block
3. Third degree AV block (complete heart block)

In *first degree AV block* all atrial impulses are conducted to the ventricles but conduction is abnormally slow, so that the PR interval is longer than .20 second. Figure 2-3 is a typical case of first degree AV block: every P wave is followed by a QRS complex, but the PR

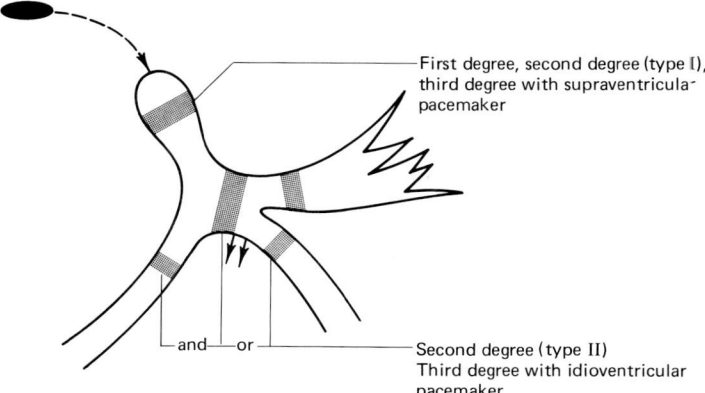

Figure 2-2. Usual location of disease producing each type of block.

interval is .32 second. First degree AV block is usually caused by conditions affecting the AV node, the most important of which are digitalis intoxication (Chapter 6), acute inferior wall myocardial infarction (Chapter 4), acute rheumatic fever and other forms of *myocarditis* (inflammation of the myocardium) and recent open heart surgery. First degree AV block does not interfere with the heart's function and, therefore, requires no treatment, but may be an important clue in diagnosis.

In *second degree AV block* some atrial impulses are conducted to the ventricles while others are blocked. Second degree AV block may be caused by diseases that affect the AV node or the bundle branches. The PR interval is not necessarily prolonged in second degree block— it may be normal, long or variable.

After second degree AV block has been diagnosed, it must be further classified as type I or type II.

In *type I second degree AV block* the PR interval changes. In a classic example such as that shown in Figure 2-4 each PR interval is a little bit longer than the previous PR, but the increase is less than the previous one so that the RR intervals become shorter until at last a P wave fails to be conducted. This is known as the *Wenckebach phenom-*

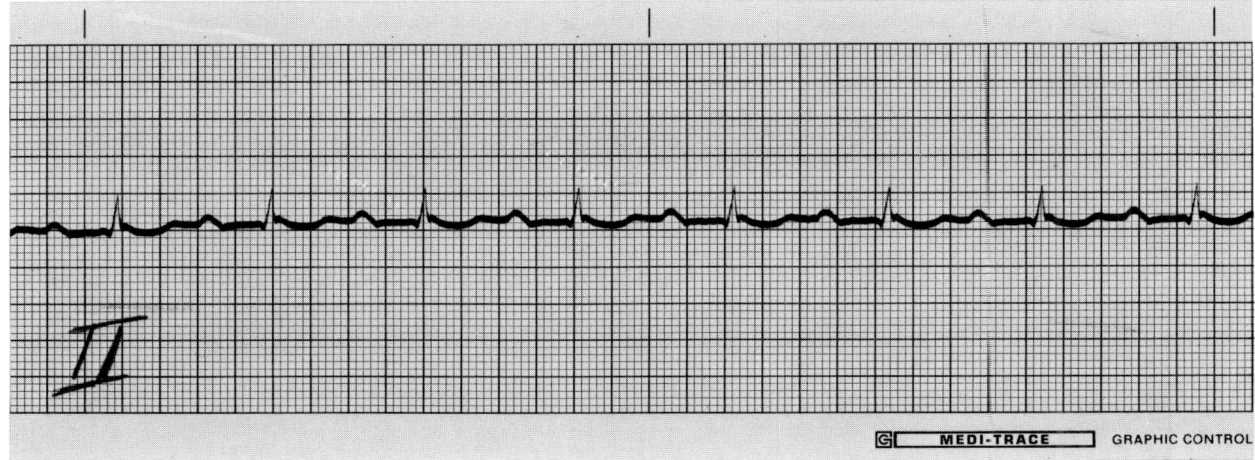

Figure 2-3.

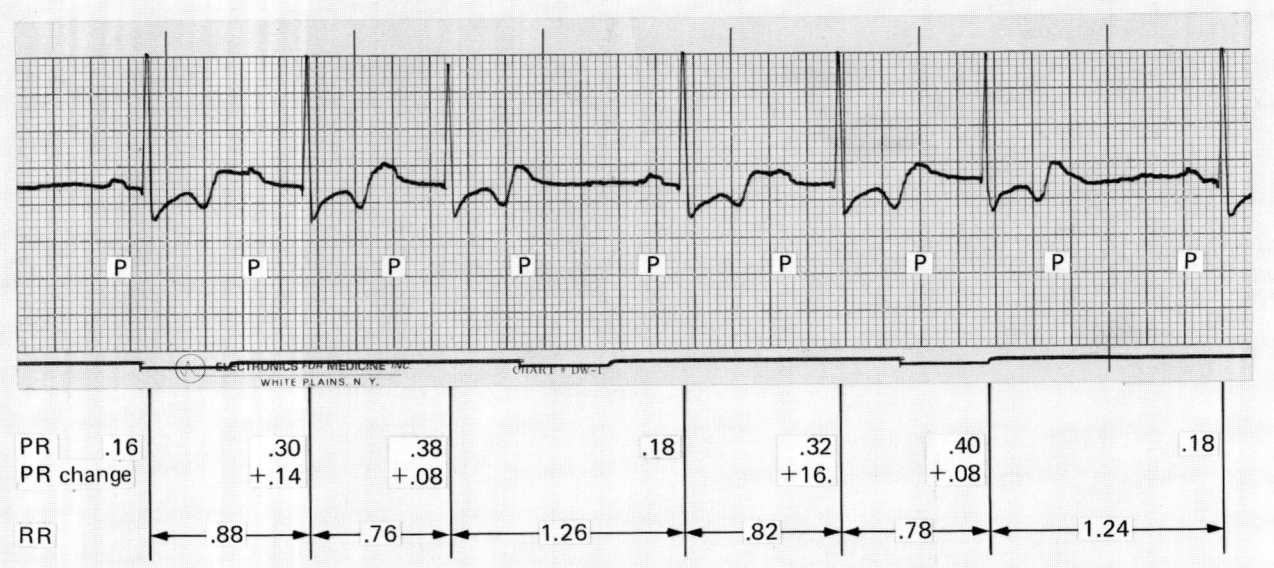

Figure 2-4.

enon. Type I second degree AV block need not be a classical Wenckebach phenomenon, however. What is essential for the diagnosis is a second degree AV block with a changing PR interval. Another important characteristic is a regular atrial rhythm plus a slower, irregular ventricular rhythm. If the PR intervals change but both rhythms are regular, then *AV dissociation* (independent beating of the atria and ventricles) is the correct diagnosis, not second degree AV block. Type I second degree block almost always means disease of the AV node, and the causes are the same as those of first degree AV block, the most important being digitalis intoxication, acute inferior myocardial infarction, myocarditis and recent heart surgery.

Type II second degree AV block is much less common than type I, but at the same time it is much more serious because it results from block in the bundle branches. Type II second degree AV block should be diagnosed when the PR intervals remain constant until one P wave is blocked, provided that at least two consecutive P waves are conducted before one is blocked. Because the PR intervals do not change, the RR intervals also do not change until there is a blocked P wave; then the RR interval will be double the usual RR interval. Bundle branch block usually accompanies type II second degree AV block, and although it occasionally happens, it is very unusual to see type II block in a patient with QRS complexes of normal duration (up to .10 second). Apparent type II second degree AV block without bundle branch block usually turns out, on closer inspection, really to be a type I block or some other less serious condition (nonconducted atrial premature beats, for example) masquerading as type II block. Because true type II block represents an advanced form of disease of the His-Purkinje system, pacemaker therapy is usually indicated.

Figures 2-4 and 2-5 are examples of type I and II second degree AV block to emphasize the differences between the two. In Figure 2-4, a monitor lead rhythm strip showing the Wenckebach phenomenon,

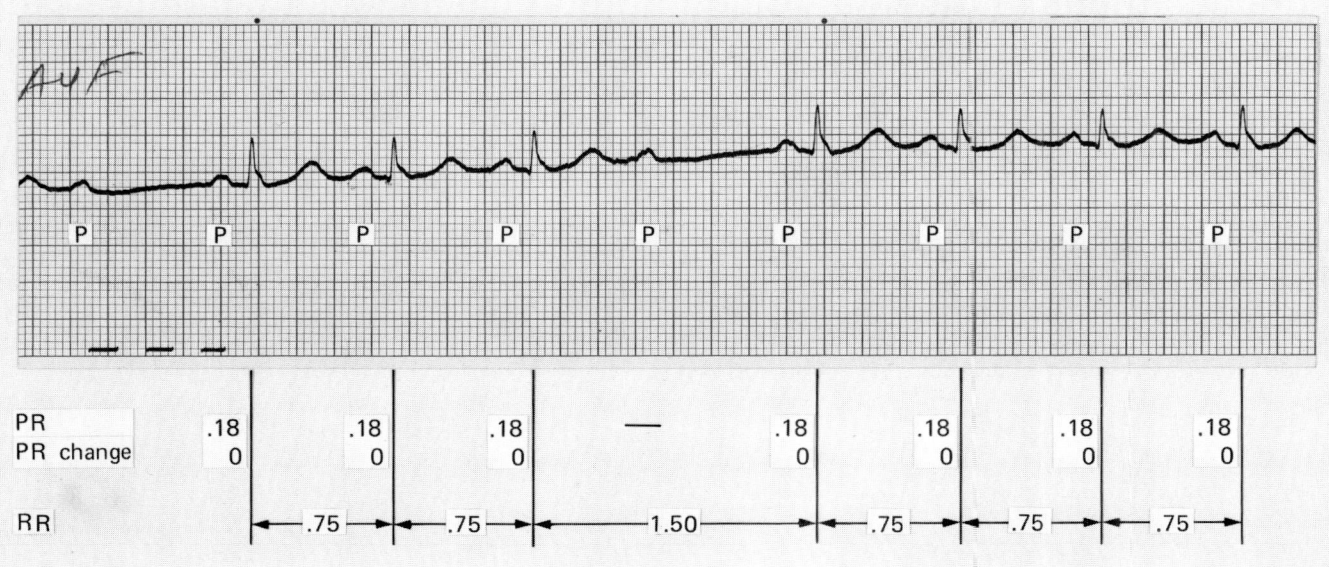

Figure 2-5.

there is a regular atrial rate of 85 per minute. The first, second, third, fifth, sixth, seventh and ninth P waves are conducted to the ventricles, while the fourth and eighth P waves are blocked: they are not followed by QRS complexes. In each group of conducted beats there is a gradual PR prolongation until the blocked P wave. Because the PR interval before the blocked beat is always the longest, and the one after it is always the shortest, the RR interval around the blocked P is *always less than twice any other RR interval on the strip.*

Figure 2-5 shows lead F from a case of type II second degree AV block. There is a regular atrial rate of 80 per minute. The first and fifth P waves are blocked; all the others are conducted with the same PR interval (.18 second). Because the PR interval is constant and the atrial rate is regular, the RR interval is also constant, except around the blocked P wave, when it is precisely double the other RR intervals. Notice, too, the wide QRS complexes (.13 second), which in other leads showed a clear bundle branch block pattern. Table 2-1 summarizes the differences between the two types of second degree AV block.

Second degree AV blocks are frequently described in terms of the *ratio* (proportion) of atrial beats to ventricular beats. For example, in Figure 2-4 every fourth P wave is blocked, so that there are four P waves for every three QRS complexes, and it would be a case of 4:3 block. In type I block, higher ratios (7:6 or 6:5) usually indicate a less serious block than ratios such as 3:2. Type II block, however, is very serious no matter what the ratio is.

2:1 AV block is a special situation that cannot properly be called type I or type II. The PR interval of the conducted beats is usually constant in 2:1 block; but since every other P wave is blocked, the diagnostic criteria for type II block (two consecutive P waves conducted) cannot be met. At the same time, a constant PR interval does

Table 2-1. Second Degree AV Block

	Type I	Type II
Location of lesion:	AV node	His-Purkinje system
PR interval of conducted beats:	Varies	Constant
RR interval:	Varies	Constant except around blocked P
RR interval around blocked P:	Less than twice the shortest RR	Exactly twice the usual RR
QRS duration:	Often normal	Usually widened (bundle branch block pattern)
Prognosis:	Often temporary	Usually persistent
Need for pacemaker:	Occasionally	Almost always

not allow a diagnosis of type I block. Only when the ratio changes to 3:2 or some other multiple can a definite classification be made.

Third Degree AV Block and Escape Beats

In complete heart block, no atrial impulses reach the ventricles. Fortunately, the sinoatrial node is not the only pacemaker in the heart. If it were, complete heart block, any disease that caused the SA node not to fire or any advanced degree of block that prevented most or all of the sinus impulses from reaching the ventricles would be immediately fatal. There are *latent* (potential) pacemakers in many areas of the heart—in the atria, in the AV junctional tissues and within the His-Purkinje network in the ventricles—whose main purpose is to stimulate the heart to beat in the event that the sinoatrial impulses do not arrive. These latent pacemakers are cells which can periodically depolarize themselves and in the process emit enough electric current to stimulate adjoining cells and trigger an impulse that can be conducted throughout the heart, just like a normal, sinoatrial impulse.

In an otherwise normal heart, these latent pacemakers are capable of depolarizing 30 to 60 times a minute. However, they do not cause the heart to beat, because their rates are slower than that of the sinoatrial node. As a result, the latent pacemakers are depolarized and reset by the arriving sinoatrial impulses before they have a chance to fire themselves. Imagine a clock that can ring every hour on the hour. If, every 45 minutes the clock is set back to one minute after the previous hour, it will never ring. On the other hand, if no one resets the clock for 60 minutes, it will ring. Likewise, a latent pacemaker will fire only when it has not been depolarized by an impulse coming from elsewhere in the heart.

When a latent pacemaker depolarizes because it has not been depolarized in time by a sinoatrial impulse, the result is an *escape beat*. Pacemakers in the atria and AV junctional tissues (collectively called *supraventricular*, above the ventricles) have more rapid rates, and are much more dependable than those in the ventricles. Supraventricular escape beats have the same or nearly the same QRS configuration as

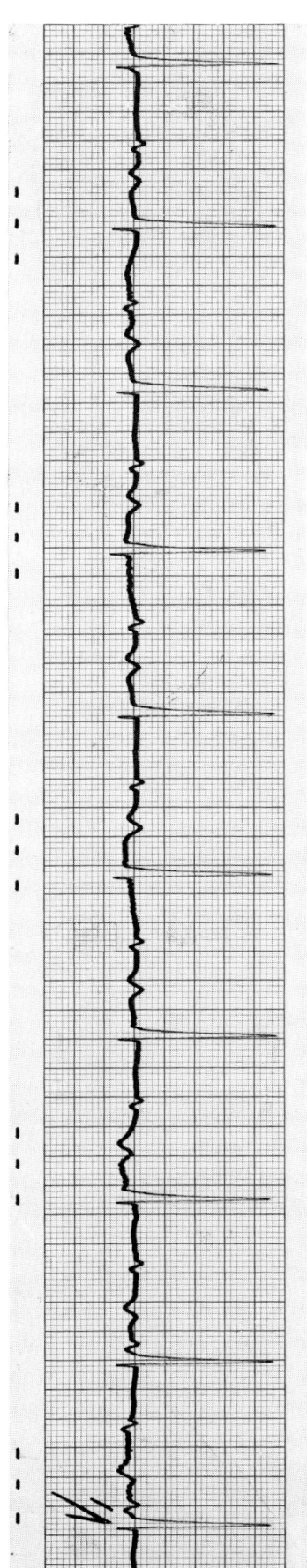

Figure 2-6.

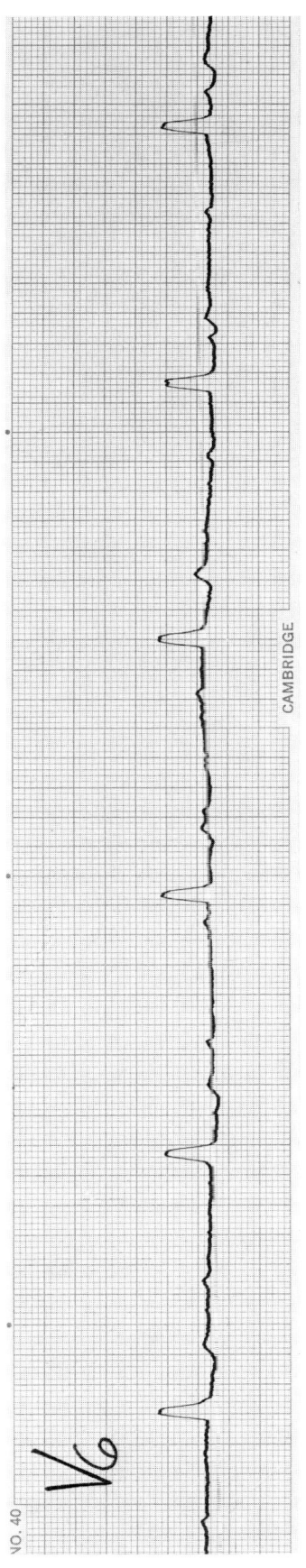

Figure 2-7.

sinoatrial beats because the impulses enter the conduction system above the branching of the Bundle of His and then are conducted into the ventricles in a relatively normal fashion. By contrast, ventricular (or *idioventricular*, literally the ventricle itself) escape beats have a bundle branch block configuration which looks different from the patient's pre-heart block QRS complexes.

Idioventricular rhythms are frequently unstable; so patients with idioventricular rhythms usually require an artificial pacemaker to prevent fainting spells or sudden death.

Third degree AV block is distinguished from other types of AV dissociation because in complete heart block (1) the atrial rate is faster than the ventricular rate and (2) the escaping pacemaker is not abnormally accelerated—i.e., the rate is less than 60 beats a minute for a junctional pacemaker and less than 45 for an idioventricular pacemaker. In some cases the escape rate is much slower, 30, 20 or even less. If the escape pacemaker is unstable, or if more than one pacemaker is firing, the ventricular rhythm may be irregular.

Figure 2-6 is a lead V_1 rhythm strip showing an example of complete heart block caused by AV nodal disease. There is a regular atrial rate of 110 per minute. Don't be fooled because some of the P waves are hidden by QRS complexes. Two consecutive P waves can be seen between the first and second and between the second and third QRS complexes. The QRS complexes are also regular at 54 per minute and of normal duration (.10 second), indicating an AV junctional escape rhythm.

By contrast, Figure 2-7 is a V_6 rhythm strip from a patient with complete heart block caused by bundle branch disease. Here, the atrial rate is 75 per minute and the ventricular rate, also regular, is 34 per minute. The slow ventricular escape rate and the wide (.13 second) QRS complexes that look different from the patient's QRS complexes before she went into complete heart block indicate that this is an idioventricular escape rhythm.

INTRAVENTRICULAR BLOCK

Intraventricular blocks are caused by *lesions* (areas of tissue damage or loss of function) in the His-Purkinje system that impair or block con-

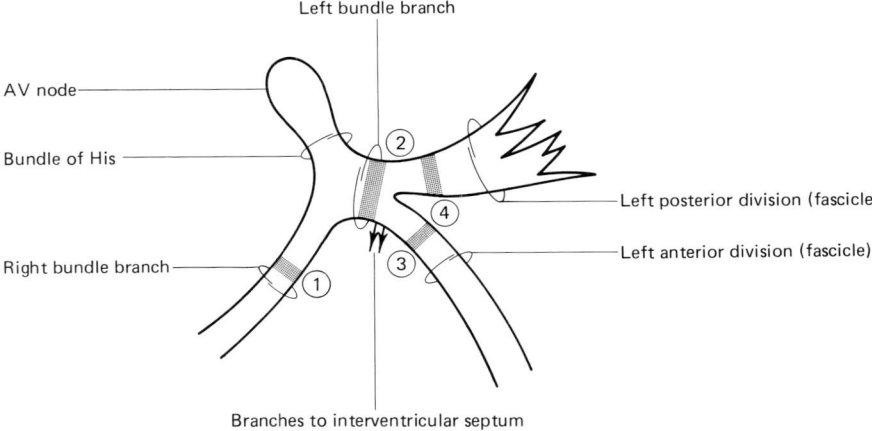

Figure 2-8.

duction in one or more of the fascicles. Figure 2-8 shows four common sites of intraventricular block. These are not the only possible sites of block; a partial lesion of the Bundle of His, for example, might only damage fibers going into the left anterior fascicle, and the resulting electrocardiogram would be indistinguishable from that resulting from a block at "3" in Figure 2-8. However, despite the oversimplification of the diagram in Figure 2-8, and even the notion of a trifascicular conducting system, the trifascicular scheme remains a valuable and generally accurate way to analyze conduction and conduction disorders within the ventricles.

Right Bundle Branch Block

Because of its long, slender structure, the right bundle branch is very vulnerable to injury. By the same token, because only a small but strategically located lesion such as "1" in Figures 2-8 and 2-9 can cause right bundle branch block, it is not uncommon to find right bundle branch block in patients without any other evidence of heart disease. When the right bundle branch cannot conduct impulses coming from the AV node, they must travel down the left bundle and cross the interventricular septum in order to enter the right ventricular Purkinje network below the zone of block, as shown by the dotted line in Figure 2-9. Thus there is a delay in right ventricular depolarization, which is best appreciated in lead V_1, the lead most sensitive to right ventricular events. The QRS is widened to at least .12 second, and a delayed, wide R wave in lead V_1 reflects the delayed right ventricular depolarization.

Figure 2-10 contrasts lead V_1 recorded from a patient with normal intraventricular conduction (*A*) with lead V_1 recorded from five different patients with right bundle branch block. In lead V_1 right bundle branch block may appear as an RSR' pattern (*B* and *D*), a QR pattern (*C*) or a wide, notched R wave (*E* and *F*); but the delayed wide R wave is the common feature of all three.

Incomplete right bundle branch block is diagnosed when V_1 displays one of these patterns, but the QRS duration is only .10 or .11 second.

Since left ventricular depolarization is normal in right bundle branch block, there is no difficulty diagnosing any coexistant left ventricular disease. In Figure 2-11, recorded from an otherwise healthy man with right bundle branch block, leads I, L and the left precordial

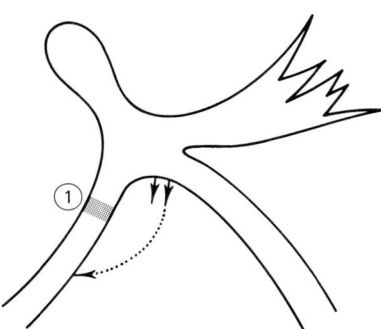

Figure 2-9. Location of block (shaded) and path of impulse (dotted line) in **right bundle branch block.**

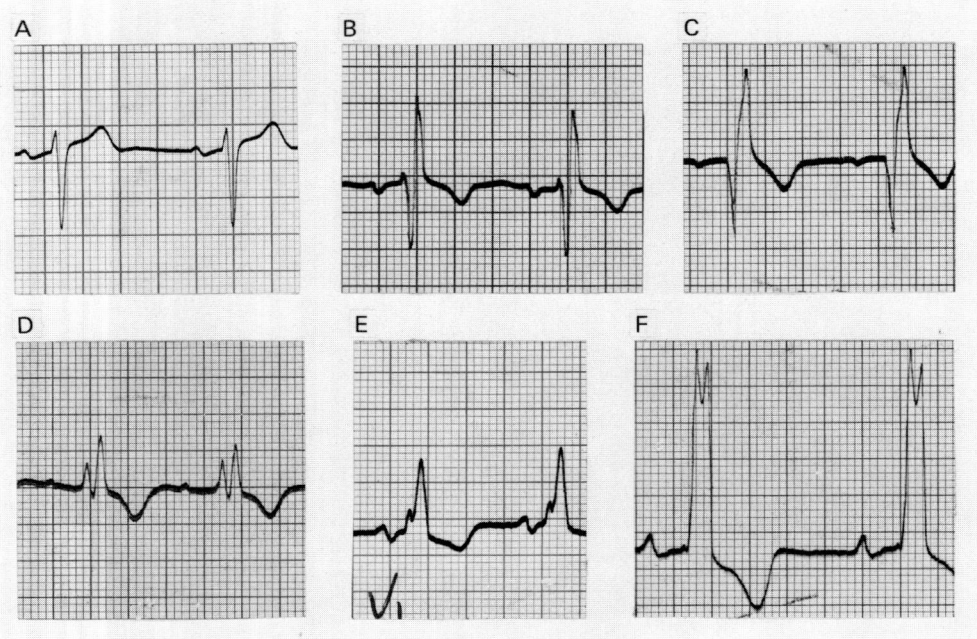

Figure 2-10.

leads all show perfectly normal R waves and small septal Q waves, as expected in the absence of left ventricular disease. Also notice that leads I, L and V_6, which look at the left side of the heart, see right ventricular currents flowing away from them and so record a wide S wave, corresponding to the wide R' in V_1. The frontal QRS axis is normal, as it should be in an uncomplicated right bundle branch block.

Left Bundle Branch Block

The left bundle branch is a rather thick structure, so a relatively large lesion is required to block it. For this reason, left bundle branch block usually means serious underlying heart disease. When the left bundle is blocked by a lesion at "2" in Figures 2-8 and 2-12, impulses must cross the interventricular septum from right to left, entering the left ventricular Purkinje network below the level of the block. There is thus a delay in left ventricular depolarization, so that the QRS is widened to at least .12 second and often more, and a broad, wide R wave is recorded in V_6, as well as leads I and L. Lead V_1, facing the right ventricle, shows either a small R and deep, wide S or else a QS. Since the Purkinje branches which cause early depolarization of the interventricular septum are branches of the left bundle, these fibers are also blocked. As a result, the septum depolarizes from right to left (opposite from the normal direction), and a septal Q wave is not recorded in leads I, L and V_6. These features can be seen in Figure 2-13, a typical case of left bundle branch block. The QRS duration is prolonged to .14 second, and wide, *slurred* (not as sharp as usual) R waves are seen in leads I, L and V_6; septal Q waves are absent. As expected in an uncomplicated case of left bundle branch block, the mean frontal axis is normal. Depressed ST segments and inverted T waves are seen in leads with large R waves. These abnormalities are expected in left bundle

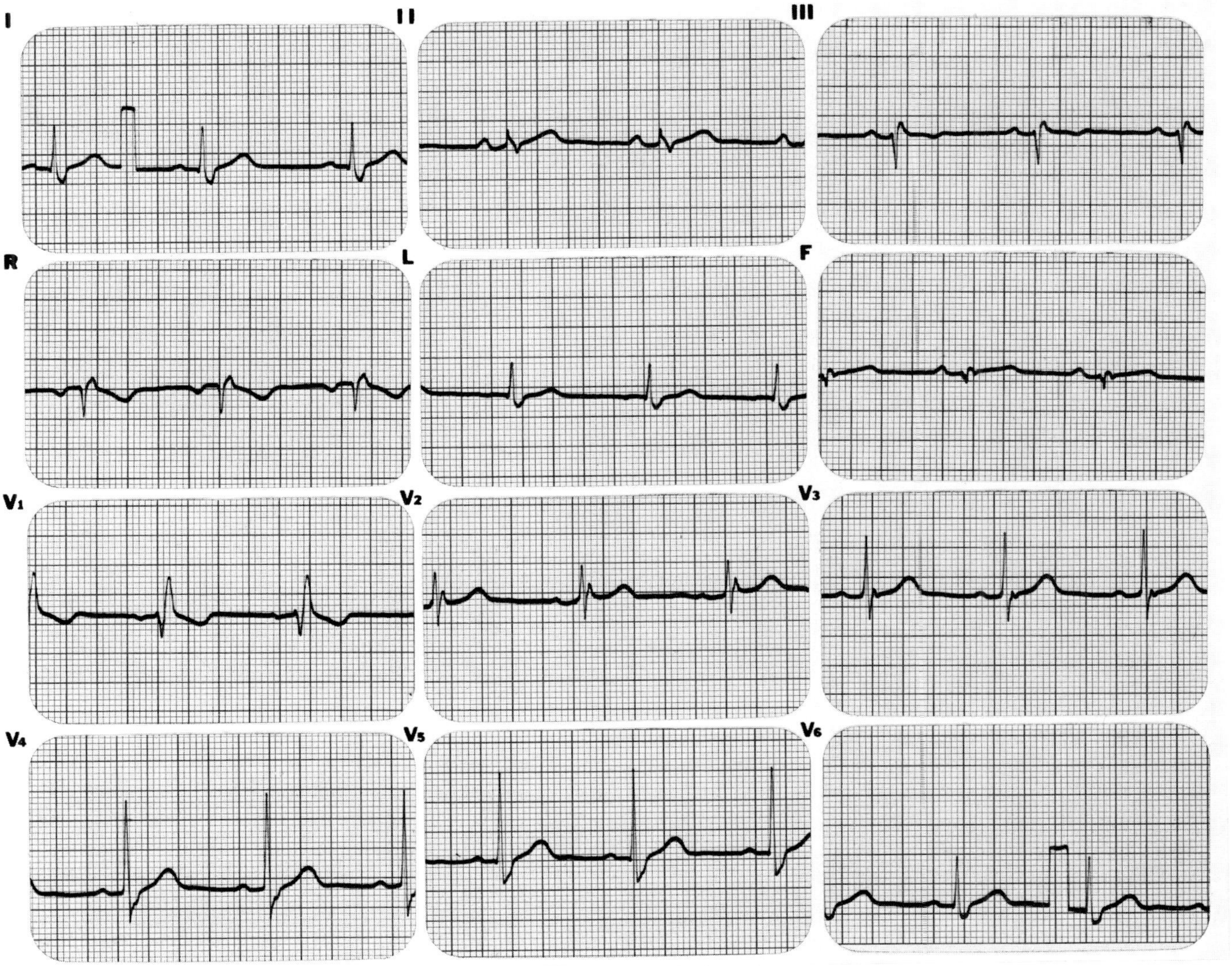

Figure 2-11.

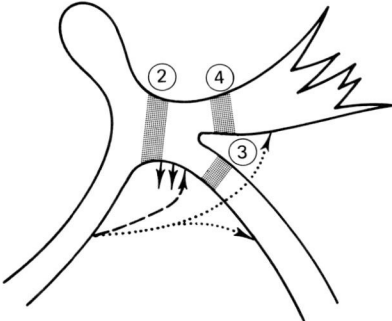

Figure 2-12. Location of block in typical ("2") and atypical ("3" and "4") left bundle branch block, and path of impulse in typical (- - -) and atypical (· · ·) left bundle branch block.

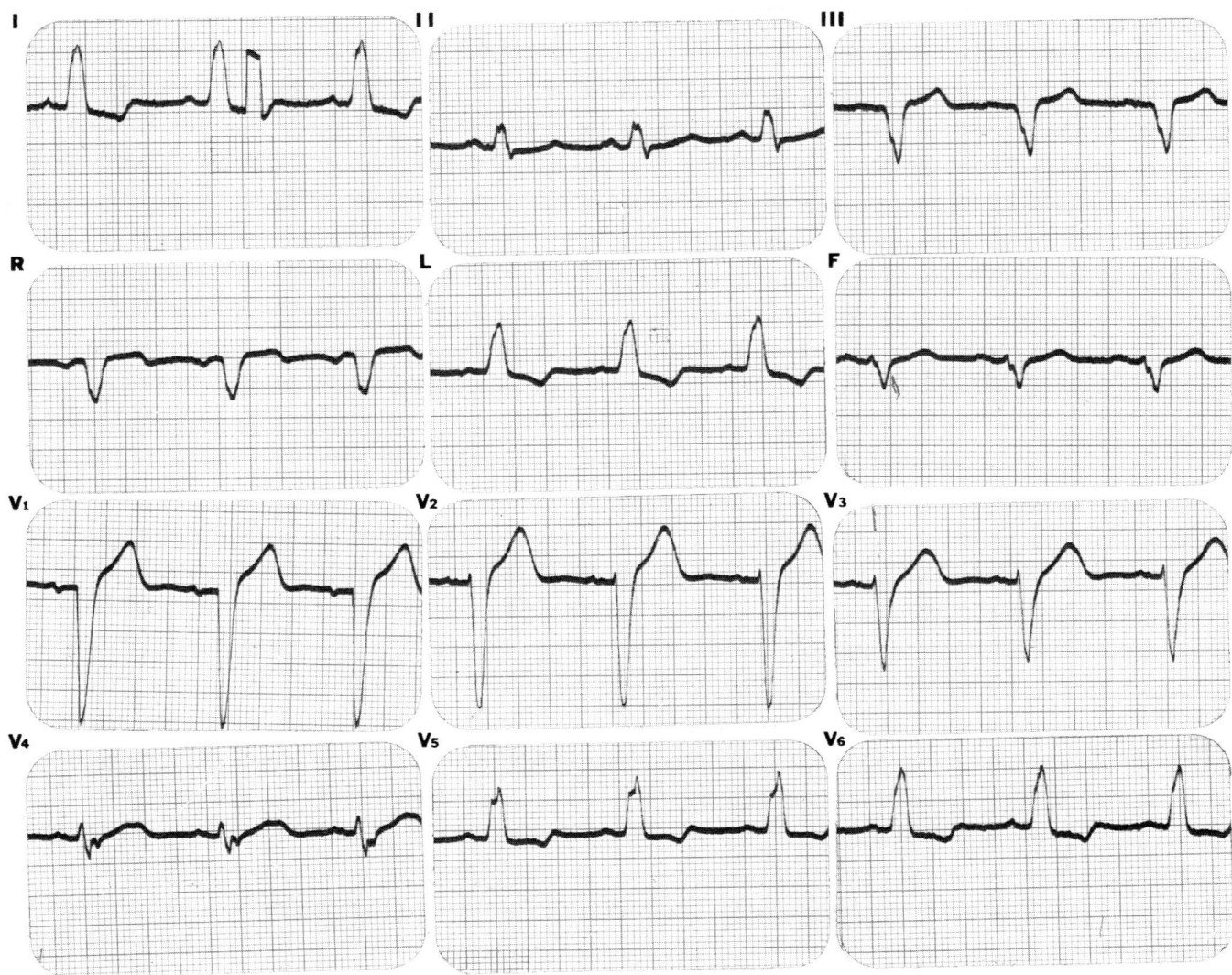

Figure 2-13.

branch block, and cannot be used to diagnose any other myocardial disease. Indeed, the abnormal QRS complexes of typical left bundle branch block so distort the usual pattern of left ventricular depolarization that it is almost impossible to make an electrocardiographic diagnosis of any associated myocardial disease.

Simultaneous block of the anterior and posterior fascicles of the left bundle (blocks "3" and "4" in Figures 2-8 and 2-12) will also cause a left bundle branch block pattern, but with one important difference from that caused by block of the main left bundle. Since sinoatrial impulses are conducted more or less normally up to points "3" and "4," the branches to the interventricular septum receive the impulses on time, and as a result the septum is depolarized normally, that is, from left to right. Therefore, a septal Q wave will be recorded in leads I, L and V_6. The pattern of left bundle branch block plus a septal Q wave is called *atypical left bundle branch block*. Since an even larger lesion is

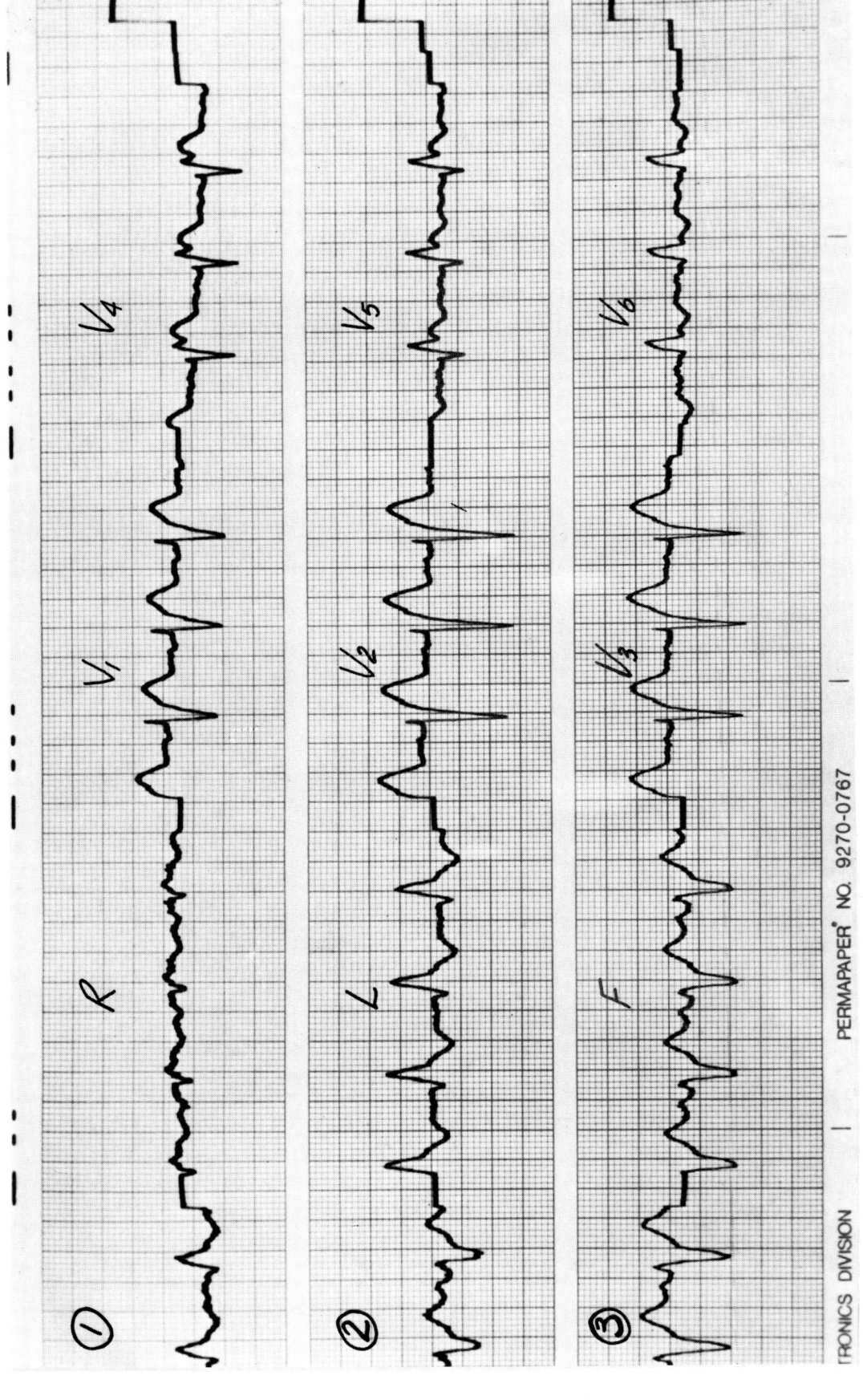

Figure 2-14.

required to block both anterior and posterior fascicles simultaneously, atypical left bundle branch block implies very extensive septal damage. Most of the time, this means anteroseptal myocardial infarction (Chapter 4). Figure 2-14 is an example of atypical left bundle branch block caused by myocardial infarction. Leads I, L and V_6 show wide, slurred R waves just like those in Figure 2-13, but the difference is that a Q wave is also present.

Left Anterior and Posterior Fascicular Block (Hemiblocks)

Uncomplicated block of either of the two main fascicles of the left bundle causes only a slight prolongation of left ventricular depolarization so that the QRS duration is usually only .10 to .12 second long. The main effect is on the sequence and, therefore, the direction of left ventricular depolarization. These changes are best appreciated in the frontal plane leads, particularly since block of either division may cause similar changes in the precordial leads, namely, a deepening of the S wave in V_5 and V_6.

The left anterior fascicle supplies the anterior and superior portions of the left ventricle. Therefore, in *left anterior hemiblock* the upper part of the left ventricle is the last part to depolarize, causing a superior shift of the mean frontal axis and abnormal left axis deviation. S is larger than R in leads II, III and F, and a large R wave is recorded in I and L. The R wave in L is often slightly slurred, reflecting the slowed intraventricular conduction, and the septal Q wave remains or even enlarges a bit in I and L. Do not make a diagnosis of left anterior hemiblock unless both a septal Q wave and abnormal left axis deviation are present. Figure 2-15 diagrams the path of left ventricular repolarization in left anterior hemiblock, and Figure 2-16 is a typical example. Notice the abnormal left axis deviation, the small R, deep S patterns in leads II, III and F, the Q waves in leads I and L and the deep S waves in leads V_5 and V_6.

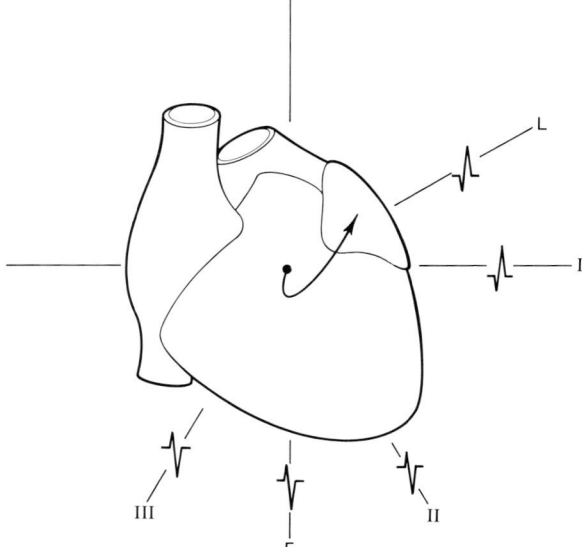

Figure 2-15. Left ventricular depolarization in left anterior hemiblock.

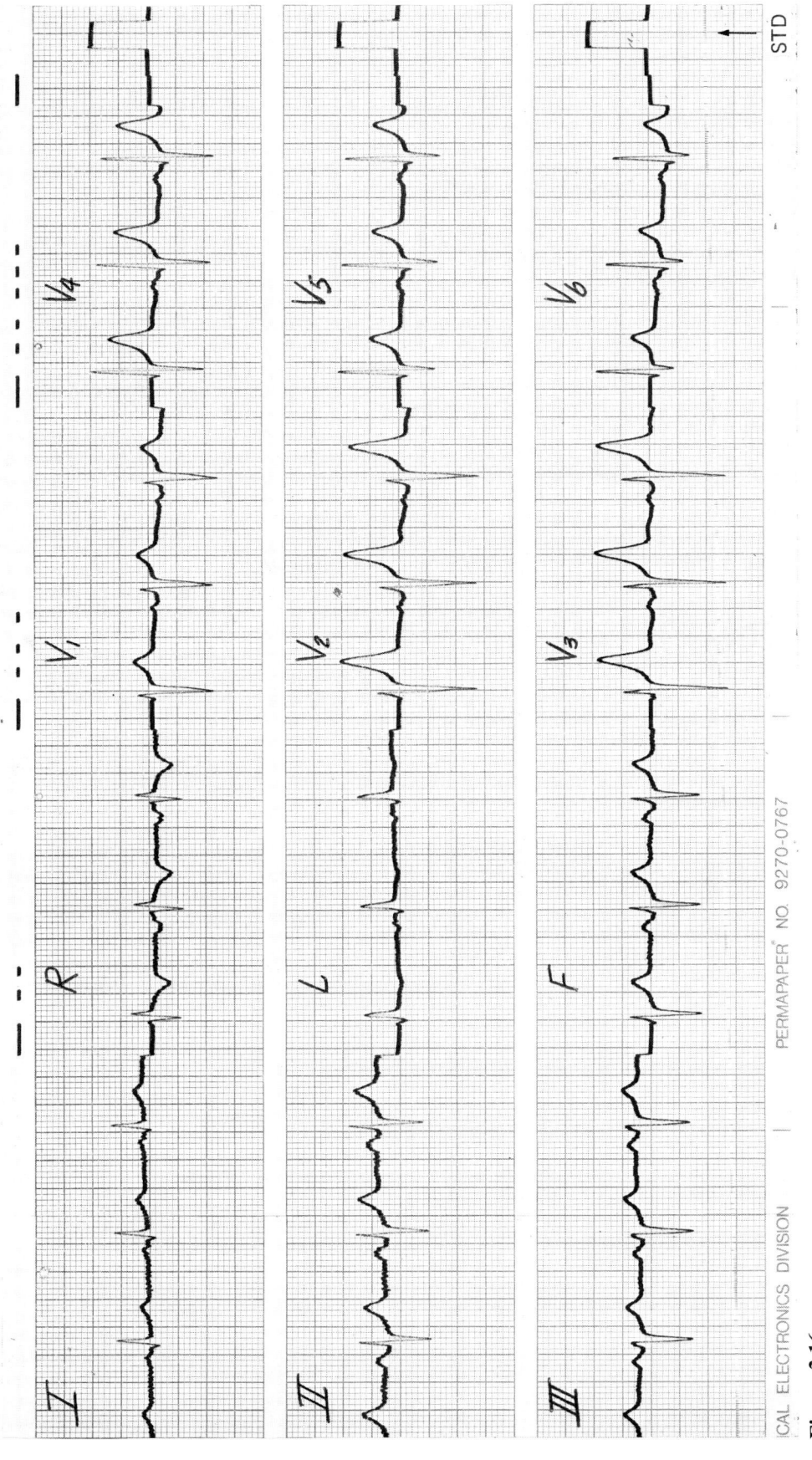

Figure 2-16.

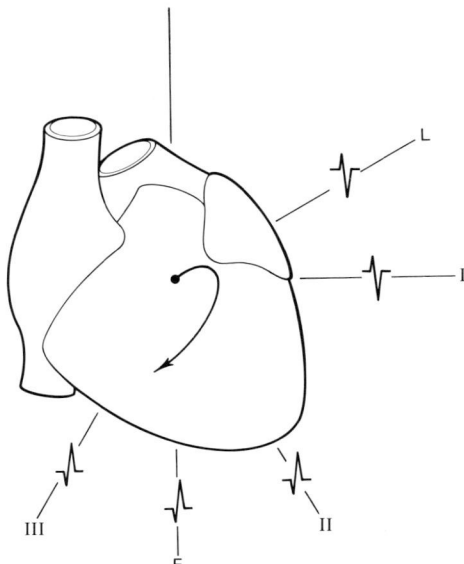

Figure 2-17. Left ventricular depolarization in left posterior hemiblock.

Left posterior hemiblock causes the inferior part of the left ventricle to depolarize last, and the resulting QRS pattern is more or less opposite to that of left anterior hemiblock. Left posterior hemiblock is diagrammed in Figure 2-17. Lead I shows a small R and large S wave, indicating the presence of abnormal right axis deviation, and a small Q and tall R wave are recorded in leads II, III and F. Unfortunately, this pattern may be seen in other conditions, including lateral wall infarction, right ventricular hypertrophy and emphysema, and even in some normal people with vertical hearts. Therefore, these conditions must be excluded before making a diagnosis of left posterior hemiblock. Since left posterior fascicular block often occurs together with other conduction disorders, the diagnosis can usually be made when abnormal right axis deviation and small Q and tall R waves in II, III and F occur in combination with right bundle branch block, or in a patient who has previously had left bundle branch block. Figure 2-18 was recorded from a patient whose electrocardiograms had previously shown left bundle branch block. Now the wide QRS complexes (.16 second) show an RSR' pattern in V_1, indicating right bundle branch block. However, abnormal right axis deviation should not be present in uncomplicated right bundle branch block. Further examination of the frontal leads shows all other the typical features of left posterior hemiblock: small R, deep S in I and L and a small Q, tall R in II, III and F, with slurring of the R waves in those leads. The exceptionally large S wave in V_6 comes from the combined effects of right bundle branch block and left posterior hemiblock.

Bifascicular and Trifascicular Block

The His-Purkinje system is often considered a trifascicular (three-branched) system consisting of the right bundle branch, and the left anterior and posterior fascicles. Since an impulse can travel from one fascicle to another beyond a zone of block, block of one or two fascicles

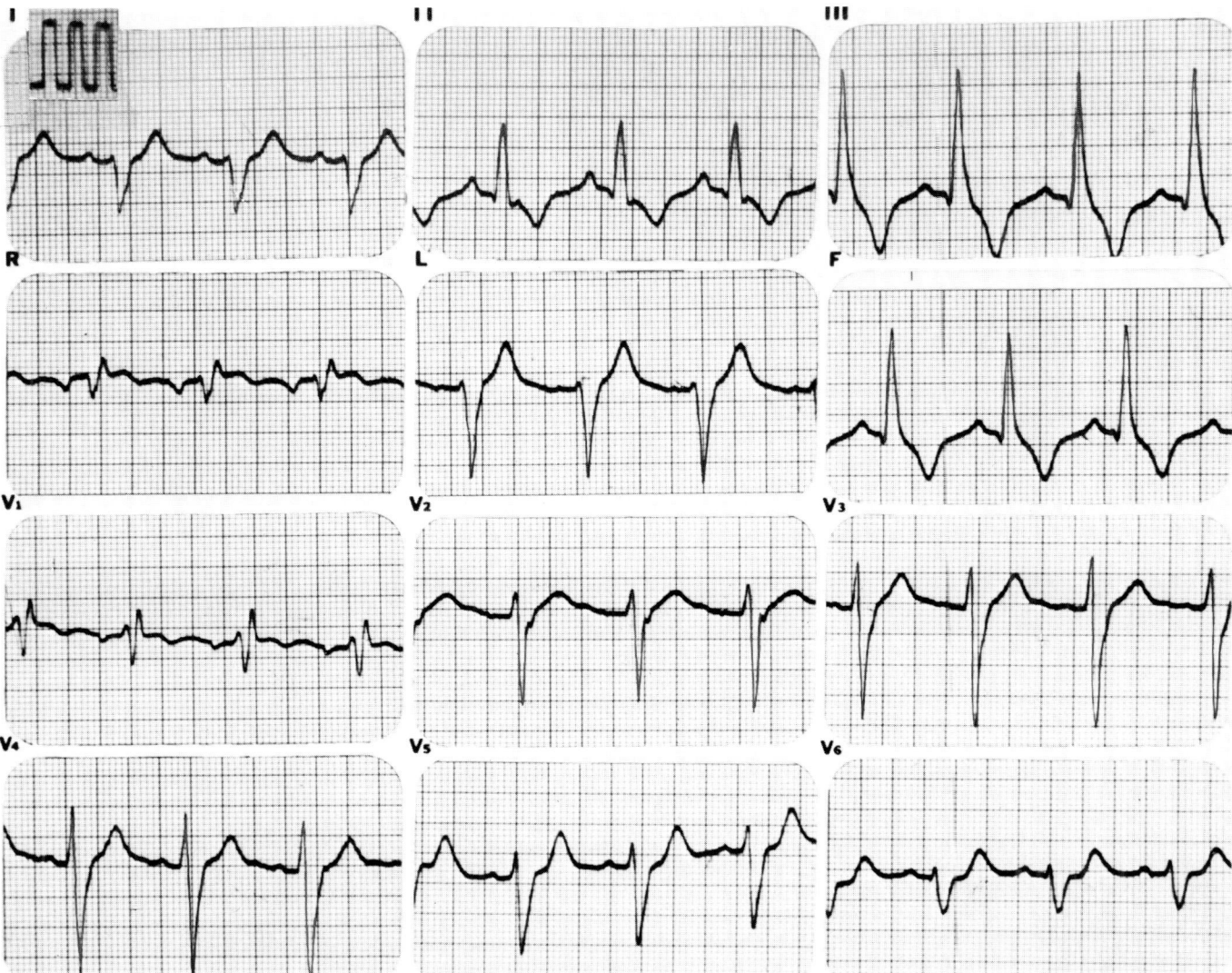

Figure 2-18.

has no significant effect on the heart's function. Complete block of all three, however, results in complete heart block.

Bifascicular block means block of any two of the fascicles, such as right bundle branch block plus left anterior or posterior fascicular block. Figure 2-19 is a typical example. The QRS duration of .14 second and the RSR′ pattern in V_1 are diagnostic of right bundle branch block. In addition, there is abnormal left axis deviation with a small R, deep S in III and F and a small Q, tall R in I and L, indicating left anterior hemiblock. Left bundle branch block is also a form of bifascicular block, since the left anterior and posterior fascicles are blocked.

Trifascicular block means abnormal conduction in all three fascicles. The block may be complete or incomplete. Incomplete trifascicular block is diagnosed when complete heart block is not present but the electrocardiographic findings indicate that none of the fas-

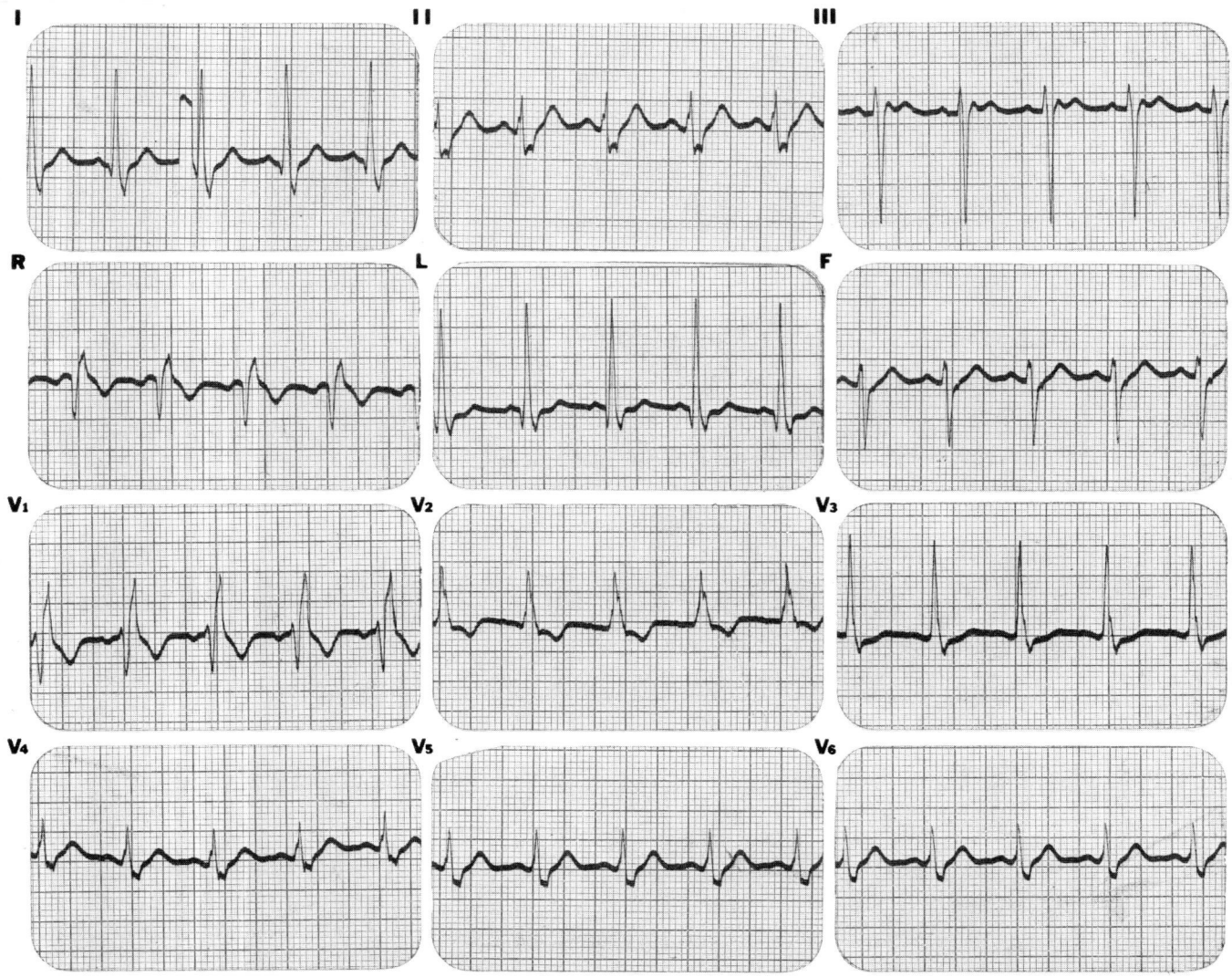

Figure 2-19.

cicles is working normally. For example, the electrocardiogram in Figure 2-18 showing left posterior hemiblock and right bundle branch block should be interpreted as showing bifascicular block. However, knowing that the patient had previously shown a left bundle branch block pattern, we can infer that the left anterior fascicle is also abnormal. Therefore, this patient has incomplete trifascicular block. Whenever a patient changes from left to right bundle branch block, or has right bundle branch block with alternating left anterior and posterior fascicular block, incomplete trifascicular block should be diagnosed. Type II second degree AV block is another form of incomplete trifascicular block.

It is often impossible to make a definite diagnosis in patients with bifascicular block plus first degree AV block. Most of the time, first degree AV block is caused by slowed conduction through the AV node; but if two fascicles are blocked and the third one conducts more

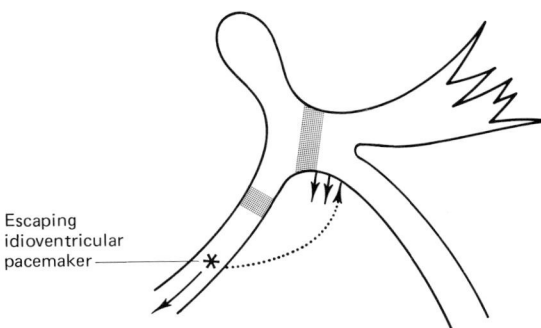

Figure 2-20.

slowly than usual, theoretically that, too, could lead to PR prolongation. Therefore, unless there is other evidence of trifascicular block, one has to hedge and diagnose "possible incomplete trifascicular block" in patients with first degree AV block who also show bifascicular block.

What makes incomplete trifascicular block so dangerous is that it indicates that the patient's last functioning fascicle is in trouble, and complete trifascicular block may soon follow, causing complete heart block. Since escaping impulses from latent supraventricular pacemakers are also prevented from reaching the ventricles, complete trifascicular block results either in complete arrest of the heart (*asystole*) or complete heart block with an idioventricular escape rhythm.

Idioventricular rhythms in complete heart block have a bundle branch block or bifascicular block pattern. If the patient had a bundle branch block before going into complete heart block, the idioventricular QRS will be different. If the escaping QRS complexes look the same as the previously conducted ones, we can infer that the impulse is proceeding along the same pathway it took before complete heart block developed, and, therefore, it must be from a supraventricular pacemaker.

Figure 2-20 explains why idioventricular rhythms have bundle branch block patterns. In this example, an escaping pacemaker in the right bundle sends its impulse rapidly and more or less normally (solid line) to the rest of the right ventricle, but the impulse has to slowly cross (dotted line) the interventricular septum just as in left bundle branch block (Figure 2-12) before it can enter the Purkinje network of the left ventricle; so the result would be an idioventricular rhythm whose QRS complexes have a left bundle branch block pattern, just like those in Figure 2-7. By the same token, if the idioventricular pacemaker were in the left main bundle, the QRS complexes would have a right bundle branch block pattern, and if it were in the left anterior fascicle, the QRS complexes might have a right bundle branch block with left posterior hemiblock pattern.

Idioventricular pacemakers are unstable and may slow or stop unexpectedly. Therefore, in cases of complete heart block caused by trifascicular block it is not uncommon to see more than one QRS pattern on the electrocardiogram, signifying a shift from one idioventricular pacemaker to another.

Chapter 3
Diagnosis of Cardiac Rhythms

The proper diagnosis of a cardiac rhythm consists of at least two words, one naming the part of the heart in which the rhythm originates and the other defining the rhythm itself. Sometimes there is a third word which describes the rhythm in greater detail. Only a limited number of words are used, but they are enough to describe all known heart rhythms. These words are listed in Table 3-1 and will be defined throughout this chapter.

To illustrate the construction of a cardiac rhythm diagnosis, consider a rapid, regular rhythm originating in the tissues of the AV junction that starts suddenly and later stops suddenly. A rapid, regular rhythm is a tachycardia. Since its origin is the AV junction, it is an AV junctional tachycardia. Because it begins and ends suddenly, it is a *paroxysmal* AV junctional tachycardia.

SINUS RHYTHMS

Under normal circumstances, the heart is under control of the sinoatrial node, and each QRS complex is preceded by a P wave which is upright in leads I, II and F and V_6. When the heart rate is between 60 and 100 beats per minute, it is called *sinus rhythm* (sometimes, regular or normal sinus rhythm). A sinus rhythm faster than 100 is called *sinus tachycardia* (tachy = fast). This is usually caused by a condition in the body requiring an increased flow of blood. No treatment is needed for the sinus tachycardia itself, but it may be a sign of another condition requiring therapy. A sinus rhythm slower than 60 beats per minute is called *sinus bradycardia* (brady = slow). Sinus bradycardia is common in young people and in well-trained athletes, but in older patients it is frequently an indication of disease of the sinoatrial node.

The sinoatrial pacemaker normally accelerates as a person breathes in and slows as he exhales. This can be a very helpful clue to dis-

Table 3-1. Terminology for Cardiac Rhythms

A. Words to define origin of rhythm
   1. Sinus
   2. Atrial
   3. AV junctional
   4. Ventricular
B. Words to define rhythm
   1. Rhythm
   2. Beat(s)
   3. Bradycardia
   4. Tachycardia
   5. Flutter
   6. Fibrillation
C. Words to describe rhythm
   1. Escape
   2. Premature
   3. Accelerated
   4. Paroxysmal
   5. Nonparoxysmal
   6. Chronic
   7. Multifocal

tinguish a rapid sinus tachycardia from the regular, ectopic supraventricular tachycardias which usually maintain a constant rate until they are about to stop. If the change is more than 10% when the slow and fast parts of the cardiogram are compared, the diagnosis is *sinus arrhythmia*. Sinus arrhythmia frequently occurs together with sinus bradycardia. Because sinus arrhythmia causes an irregular rhythm, it may be confused with other, abnormal heart rhythms. Figure 3-1 is an example of a sinus arrhythmia. The longest RR interval is 1.14 seconds and the shortest .74, corresponding to heart rates of 53 and 81 per minute. Notice the gradual speeding up and slowing down of the heart rate, corresponding to the phases of respiration, and notice, too, that the P waves all look the same.

A diseased sinoatrial node may intermittently or completely fail to emit impulses. This results in either of two similar arrhythmias, *sinoatrial block* and *sinoatrial arrest*. Although they can be differentiated by careful analysis of the electrocardiogram, practically the distinction is not very important, since either one may cause dangerous slowing of the heart. Figure 3-2 is a case of intermittent sinoatrial block. The arrows point to two places where the sinoatrial impulse fails to appear. As a result, there is no P wave or QRS, and the heart rate falls from 48 to 24 per minute.

ECTOPIC RHYTHMS

Any heart rhythm that does not arise in the sinoatrial node is an *ectopic rhythm*. There are two basic types: (1) escape beats and rhythms and (2) premature beats and tachycardias. Escape beats appear when the sinoatrial impulse is delayed or blocked so that latent pacemaker cells have an opportunity to fire; three or more consecutive escape beats are an escape rhythm. A *premature beat*

46 / **Basic Electrocardiography Handbook**

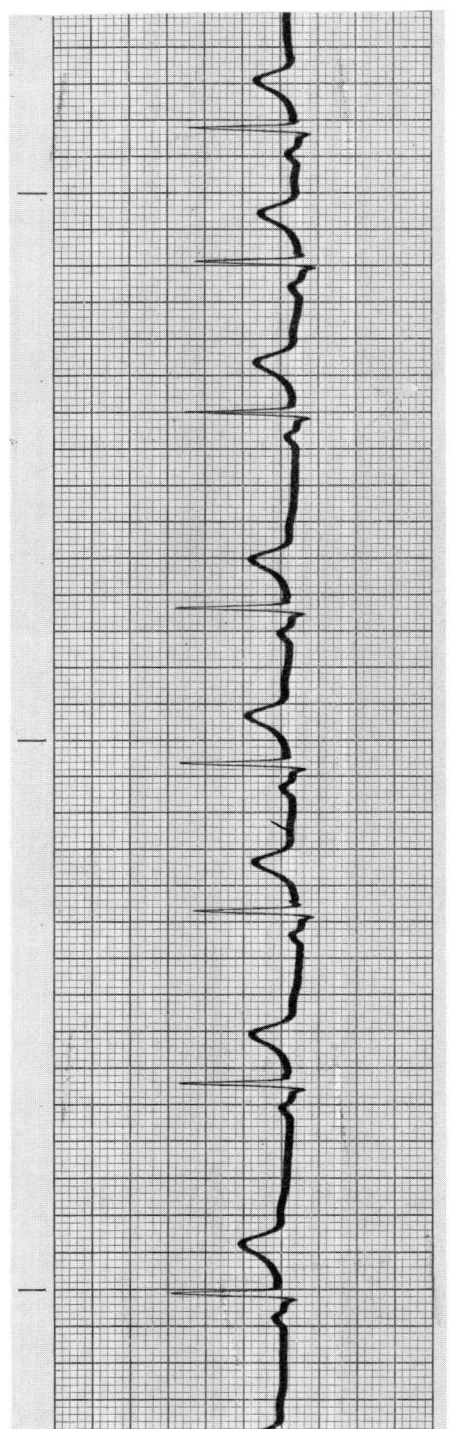

Figure 3-1.

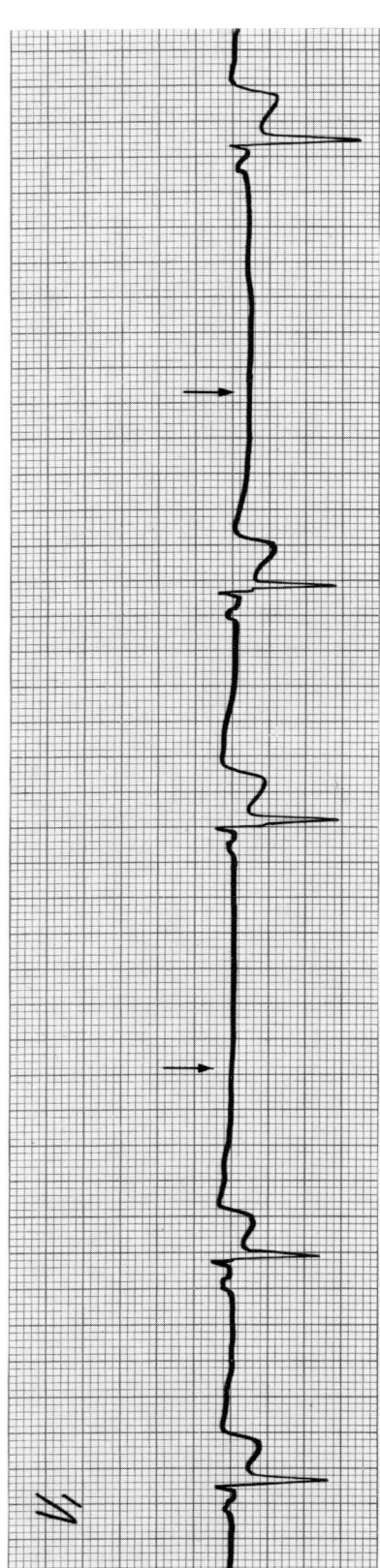

Figure 3-2.

occurs when an ectopic pacemaker fires early, before the sinoatrial impulse has a chance to reach it; two consecutive premature beats are called a *salvo*, and three or more, a tachycardia.

Once an ectopic rhythm begins, it may be sustained by one of two mechanisms. The first is repeated firing by the ectopic pacemaker cells (*automaticity*); if the rate is faster than expected for a pacemaker in that part of the heart, it is called *enhanced automaticity*. The other mechanism is *reentry*; here, a *circus movement* becomes established so that the impulse goes around and around a circuit of conducting cells.

Figure 3-3 diagrams the impulse path in a reentrant arrhythmia. In this example, there is a connection between the reentrant circuit and the AV node at point *A*. Each time the impulse comes around to point *A*, it is conducted to the AV node, from which it can be conducted to the ventricles. The effect is the same as if there were an ectopic pacemaker at point *A* firing rapidly because of enhanced automaticity. The same number of ectopic impulses would reach the AV node and the same number of QRS complexes would follow. Reentry is known to be the basic mechanism for atrial flutter and for supraventricular tachycardias in patients with preexcitation (Chapter 5), but it may be responsible for many other arrhythmias as well.

Ectopic rhythms are called *tachycardias* if the rate exceeds 100 per minute (or 70 in the case of an AV junctional rhythm). If the rhythm is not fast enough to be called a tachycardia, it is merely identified by its site of origin (atrial, junctional or idioventricular rhythm). There is a gray zone that includes rhythms that are faster than the normal escape rhythm in that part of the heart but not fast enough to be tachycardias; these rhythms are called *accelerated rhythms*. The term is used for an AV junctional rhythm between 60 and 70 beats per minute (accelerated junctional escape rhythm) or an idioventricular rhythm between 45 and 100 beats per minute (accelerated idioventricular rhythm).

Dealing with ectopic rhythms is one of the most important aspects of cardiac care. A basic principle is that the heart usually pumps

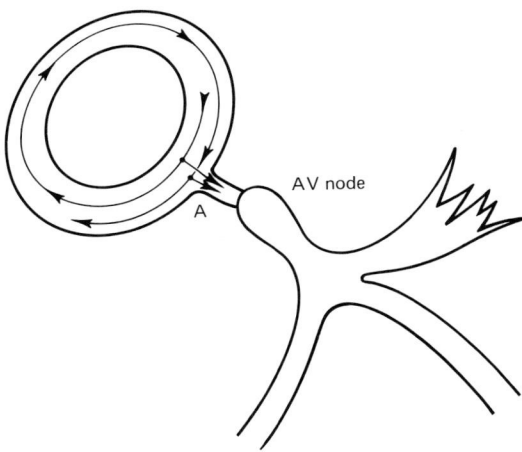

Figure 3-3.

most efficiently when it beats between 60 and 100 times a minute. Cardiac performance often suffers at rates significantly faster or slower than these limits, and the *cardiac output* (amount of blood pumped each minute) tends to fall. Therefore, even though all ectopic rhythms are abnormal, only those that are so fast or so slow that they reduce cardiac output and those that are life-threatening because they may lead to cardiac arrest require urgent treatment. Most of the time, ectopic tachycardias have to be slowed or stopped, while escape rhythms need to be speeded up. As a rule, treatment is not difficult, provided that the correct diagnosis has been made. Accelerated junctional and accelerated idioventricular rhythms usually do not require any treatment; their main importance is as a clue to the condition that caused them to appear.

PREMATURE BEATS

The simplest cardiac arrhythmias are premature beats. A premature beat is identified because it is early—it interrupts the usual regularity of a sinus rhythm. The diagnosis is completed by deducing the beat's site of origin. If the ectopic pacemaker is supraventricular, the premature QRS is usually identical to or very much like the patient's usual QRS. Supraventricular premature beats can usually be classified as atrial or junctional premature beats by examining the P wave and the PR interval.

An *atrial premature beat* (APB) arises from an atrial focus outside of the sinoatrial node; therefore, the impulse spreads through the atrium differently from a sinoatrial impulse. The result is a P wave that not only is early but also looks different from the usual P wave. It may be taller, smaller, wider or narrower; but it is different, and the difference distinguishes it from an early beat in a sinus arrhythmia. Furthermore, since the impulse of an APB passes through the entire length of the AV node, the PR interval will be the same as the patient's usual PR interval or longer, but never shorter.

Figure 3-4 is a V_1 rhythm strip in which the third, sixth and ninth beats are atrial premature beats. Notice that the patient's normal P waves are biphasic, consisting of a short positive deflection followed by a wide, shallow, negative deflection, and that the PR interval is .14 second. By contrast, the premature P waves consist of a negative deflection then a positive deflection which is a bit wider than that of the normal P, and the PR interval of the premature beats is .20 second. All the QRS complexes look the same.

The explanation for the longer PR interval after the premature P waves in this case is *relative refractoriness* of the AV node. Refractoriness is an important property of myocardial cells and conducting tissues. For most of the interval between a cell's depolarization and its repolarization, it is *absolutely refractory*. That means no matter how large an electrical signal reaches it, nothing will happen. If it is a myocardial cell, it will not contract. If it is a conducting cell, it will not conduct. For a short time before a cell becomes completely repolarized and ready again to function normally, it is relatively refractory; during this time, if it responds to an electrical impulse,

Diagnosis of Cardiac Rhythms / 49

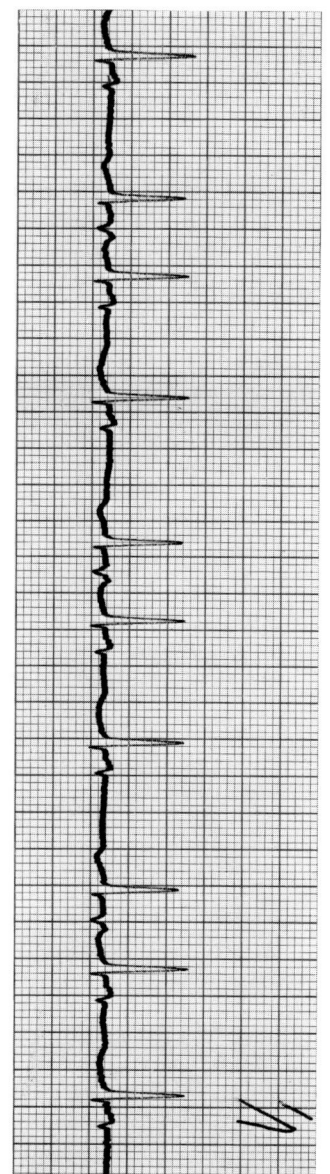

Figure 3-4.

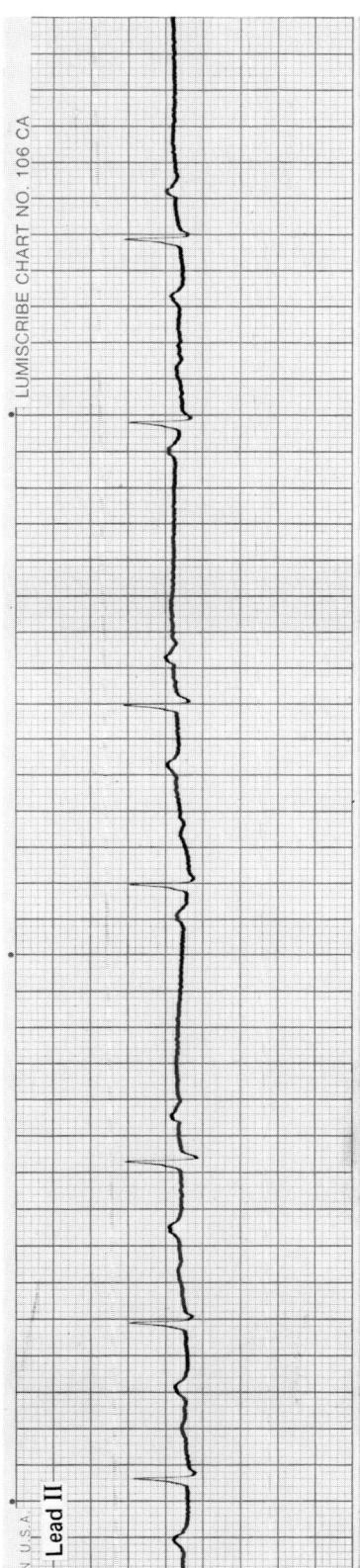

Figure 3-5.

the response is likely to be abnormal. In the case of the AV node, the result is slower conduction and, therefore, a longer PR interval.

An atrial premature beat early enough to reach the AV node during the absolute refractory period will not be conducted to the ventricles, so no QRS will follow. This is a *nonconducted* or *blocked atrial premature beat*. Since the premature atrial impulse has depolarized the atria including the SA node, a pause follows until the next sinoatrial impulse causes the heart to beat again. Blocked APB's frequently fall on the T wave of the preceding QRS complex; therefore, they are easily overlooked unless one carefully compares the T wave with another one in the same lead.

Figure 3-5 is a lead II rhythm strip in which there are long pauses after the third, fifth and seventh QRS complexes. The T waves following these QRS complexes appear larger than all the other T waves, but closer inspection reveals that these "larger T waves" are really nonconducted APB's. Always look carefully for blocked APB's when the electrocardiogram shows unexpected pauses in a sinus rhythm.

A premature atrial impulse may also encounter refractoriness in the His-Purkinje system if one or more of the fascicles has not repolarized by the time the impulse arrives. In such a case, the QRS complex that follows the premature P wave will have a fascicular block or a bundle branch block pattern. It is very important that this phenomenon (called *aberrant conduction*) be recognized, since most of the time a premature beat with a wide QRS complex is a premature ventricular beat, potentially much more serious than an aberrantly conducted supraventricular beat.

Figure 3-6 is a lead II rhythm strip showing sinus rhythm with four atrial premature beats (P'). The first and third premature P waves are earlier than the second and fourth, as indicated by their respective PP' intervals of .42 and .58 second. As a result of their greater prematurity, the first and third premature P waves are followed by longer PR intervals (.24 second) and aberrantly conducted QRS complexes. The later-arriving second and fourth premature P waves have PR intervals only slightly longer than the patient's usual ones (.20 second as opposed to .18 second) and no aberrant ventricular conduction.

Atrial premature beats may be *unifocal* (arising from one pacemaker) or *multifocal*. Unifocal APB's have the same P wave con-

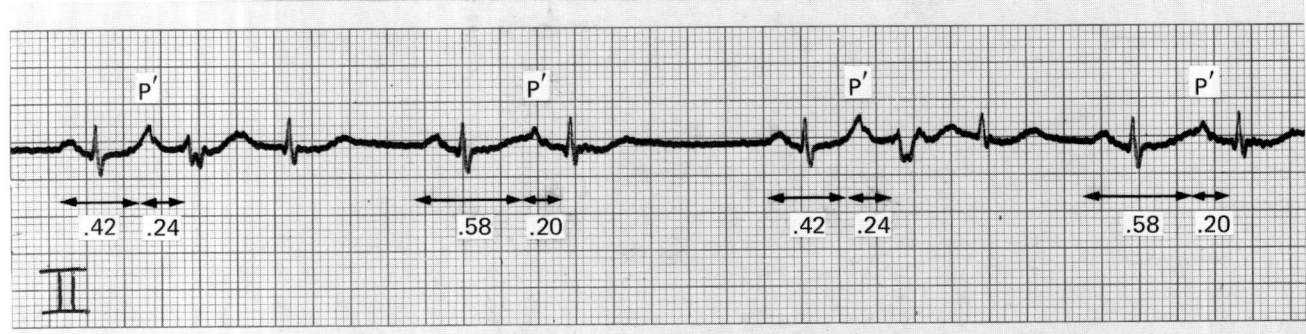

Figure 3-6.

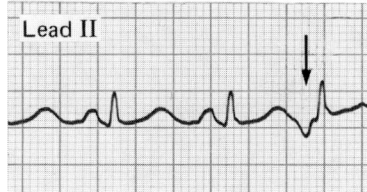

Figure 3-7.

figuration, since the impulses all arise from the same ectopic atrial pacemaker. Multifocal APB's are diagnosed when two or more ectopic P waves can be identified in the same lead.

AV junctional premature beats result from premature impulses arising in the AV junctional tissues. Pacemaker cells are located all around the AV node; when they fire, the impulse enters the AV node and is conducted in the normal *antegrade* (forward) direction to the ventricles and *retrograde* (backward) into the atria. If the impulse is not blocked in either direction, the result is a typical supraventricular QRS complex, but an inverted P wave in leads II, III and F, showing that the atrial depolarization wave has moved from the bottom up, just the opposite to its usual direction.

Figure 3-7 is a lead II rhythm strip showing a typical junctional premature beat (arrow). The QRS complex looks normal, but it is preceded by an inverted P wave with a PR interval of .11 second. When a retrograde junctional P wave precedes its QRS complex, the PR interval is almost always shorter than .12 second. Depending on the location of the junctional pacemaker, and the relative speeds of retrograde and antegrade conduction, the P wave may precede, coincide with or follow the QRS complex.

Figure 3-8 shows some beats in lead II from three different patients with junctional rhythms and retrograde conduction into the atria. In *A*, the inverted P waves precede the QRS complex with PR interval of .08 second; in *B* they coincide with the QRS, so they are invisible; and in *C* they follow the QRS with an RP interval of .08 second.

Not all junctional premature beats are identical to the patient's usual QRS complexes, however. Sometimes there is aberrant ven-

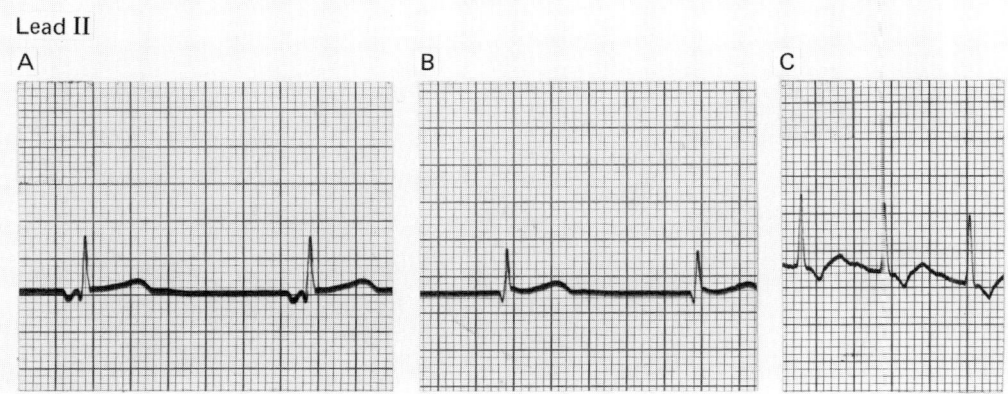

Figure 3-8.

tricular conduction caused by refractoriness of conducting tissue, just like aberrantly conducted atrial premature beats. Most of the time, and particularly when the ventricular aberration occurs at slow rates, there is another explanation, which is diagrammed in Figure 3-9. Within the Bundle of His, and probably within the AV node itself, the Purkinje fibers are grouped as they are in the fascicles. Therefore, a junctional impulse arising at *A* might reach the fibers of the left posterior fascicle just a little sooner than those of the left anterior fascicle and those of the right bundle branch. The result would be a distortion of the QRS complex, perhaps not enough to show the full characteristics of a bundle branch block or a fascicular block, but enough to make the junctional beat a bit wider than the patient's normal QRS complexes. This situation is illustrated by the rhythm strip shown in Figure 3-10, where the junctional premature beats are only a little wider than the normal beats.

Sometimes junctional premature beats occur without retrograde conduction. Although the junctional impulses tend to go up into the atria as shown by the dotted lines in Figure 3-9, they cannot do so if the atria have already been depolarized by the sinoatrial node. Figure 3-11 is a rhythm strip in which the second, fourth and eighth beats are junctional premature beats. Notice their slight aberration when compared to the normal QRS complexes. Notice, too, the normal P waves, which can be seen just after the first and third premature beats, and just before the second. The explanation is that the premature junctional impulses in this patient are conducted rapidly down to the ventricles, but only slowly upwards through the AV node. By the time they reach the upper end of the AV node (point *B*, Figure 3-9) the sinoatrial node has already depolarized the atria in the usual manner, so the retrograde junctional impulse is blocked before it can enter the atria.

Ventricular premature beats (VPB) arise from pacemaker cells below the branching of the Bundle of His. They almost always have a bundle branch block pattern and a QRS duration of at least .12 second, just like ventricular escape beats (Chapter 2). Frequently the initial deflection, either Q or R, is slurred because of slow con-

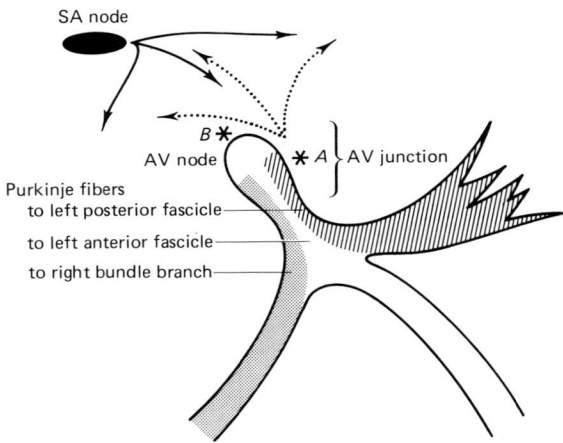

Figure 3-9.

Diagnosis of Cardiac Rhythms / 53

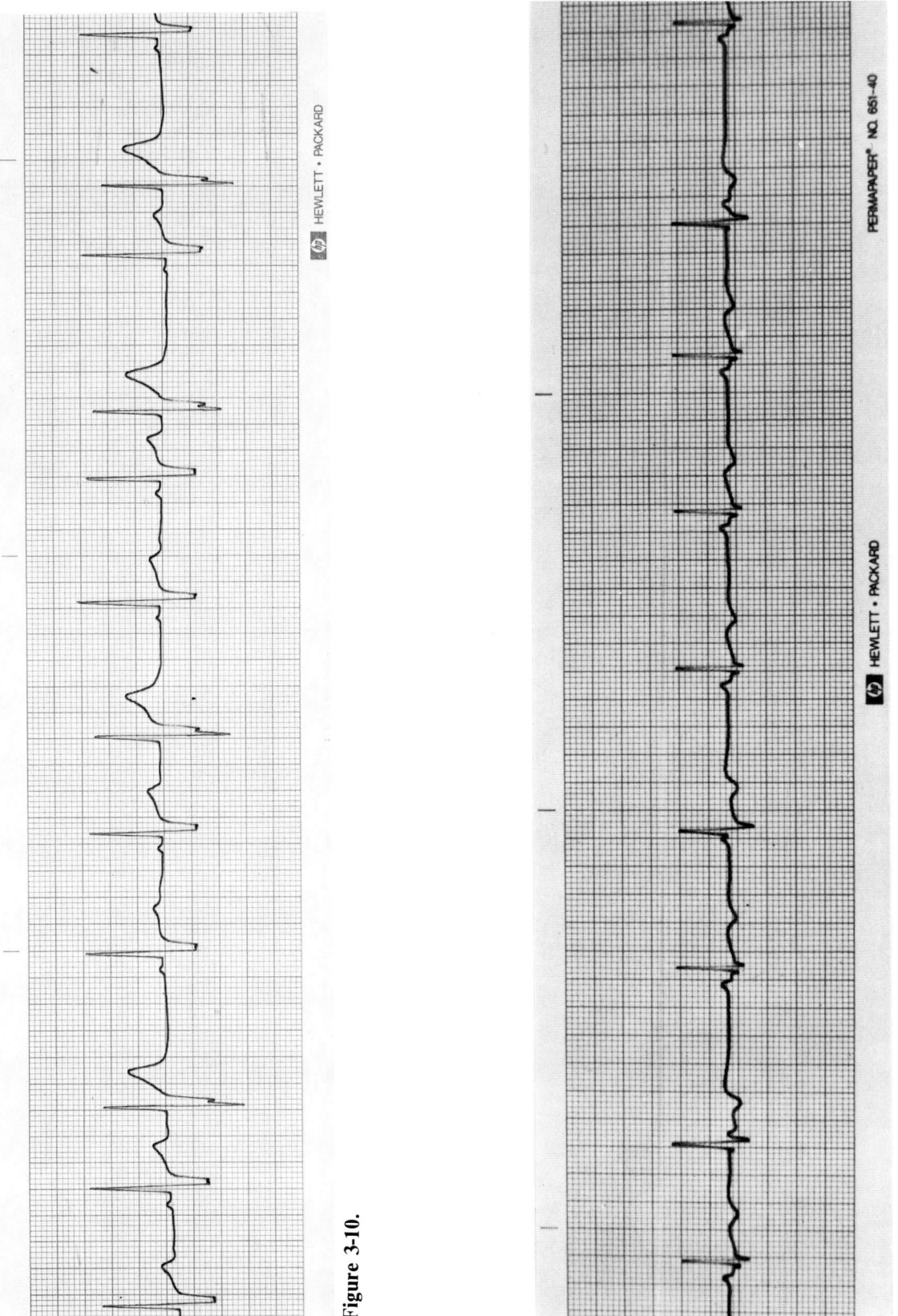

Figure 3-10.

Figure 3-11.

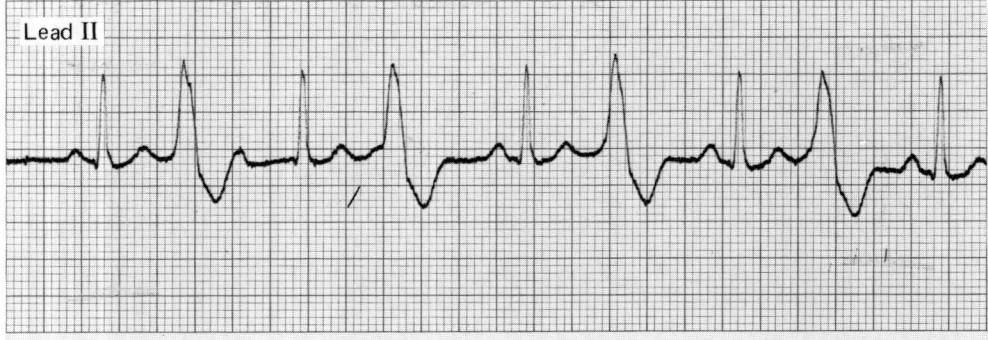

Figure 3-12.

duction of the impulse through the Purkinje branches. In any case, the QRS pattern of a VPB will be quite different from the patient's usual beats. Furthermore, VPB's are not preceded by premature P waves. Indeed, if what seems to be a VPB follows a premature P wave, then it is probably not a VPB at all but an aberrantly conducted atrial or junctional premature beat. However, it is not unusual to see a normal P before a VPB if the VPB appears relatively late in diastole. This is a chance relationship—in such cases the PR interval is shorter than normal for that patient, indicating that the ventricle was depolarized by the ectopic ventricular impulse before the normal impulse could enter the Purkinje system.

Figure 3-12 is a lead II rhythm strip in which sinus beats alternate with ventricular premature beats, easily recognizable by the absence of a preceding P wave and the wide QRS complexes (.14 second) very different from the patient's normal beats. When every other beat comes from a different focus, as in this case, it is called a *bigeminal rhythm*. This particular example is ventricular bigemini, but you may also encounter atrial bigemini, and so on.

Like APB's, VPB's may be unifocal or multifocal. Unifocal VPB's look the same, while multifocal VPB's are recognized because they have various configurations, depending on where the impulses originate. Multifocal VPB's suggest more serious ventricular disease than unifocal VPB's. Figure 3-13 is a V_5 rhythm strip that includes

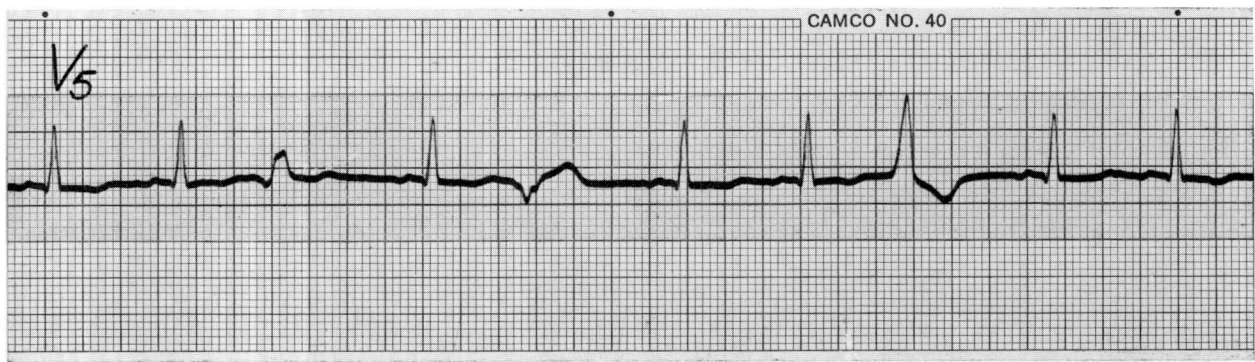

Figure 3-13.

VPB's from three different foci. All have a QRS duration of at least .12 second, and a slurred Q wave, R wave or both.

Diagnosis of Premature Beats with Wide QRS Complexes

Even though premature beats usually have little or no effect on the cardiac output, there are several important reasons why accurate diagnosis is important: (1) Premature beats mean that either there is a pacemaker with abnormally enhanced automaticity or a reentrant pathway in the part of the heart from which the beats arise. Therefore, the presence of premature beats is often an indication of disease or abnormal function in their chamber of origin. (2) The same mechanisms that cause premature beats can also cause sustained tachyarrhythmias. For example, a patient with atrial premature beats is more likely to develop atrial fibrillation or some other atrial tachyarrhythmia than one without them. Likewise, a patient with ventricular premature beats has an increased risk of developing ventricular tachycardia or fibrillation. Since ventricular arrhythmias are generally much more dangerous than supraventricular arrhythmias, the discovery of frequent ventricular premature beats might well lead to the administration of preventive treatment, while it would be only rarely indicated for supraventricular premature beats. (3) Sometimes, a patient has a paroxysmal tachycardia that defies diagnosis, and then sinus rhythm returns either spontaneously or because of a treatment such as DC shock, which can cure almost any paroxysmal tachyarrhythmia. Frequently, the patient will have premature beats, either before or after the tachycardia. By diagnosing the premature beats, we can often make a good presumptive diagnosis of the tachycardia based on "guilt by association" (this may not be a sound legal principle but it usually holds in electrocardiography). Some examples of this principle appear later in this chapter (see below, Figures 3-30 and 3-31, 3-37 and 3-38).

It is particularly important to be accurate in diagnosing ventricular premature beats, since a diagnosis of VPB's is often followed by the initiation of vigorous and potentially toxic treatment. Since ventricular premature beats have wide QRS complexes, if a beat has a QRS complex of normal duration, we don't have to worry about a ventricular origin. However, the opposite does not always hold— a premature beat with a wide QRS complex is not necessarily a VPB. There are two other possibilities: (1) If a patient has a bundle branch block or any other intraventricular conduction disorder while in sinus rhythm, then any supraventricular impulse conducted along the same path will also have a wide QRS complex. Therefore, *if a patient with a bundle branch block or any other intraventricular conduction disorder has premature beats with the same wide QRS complexes, they must be supraventricular.* (2) Aberrantly conducted supraventricular beats may also have QRS complexes whose duration is .12 second or more. If a premature P wave of atrial or junctional origin can be identified before the wide QRS complex as in Figure 3-6, again there is no difficulty with diagnosis.

The major problem in differentiating VPB's from aberrantly conducted supraventricular beats occurs when there are no visible P waves. Slurred QRS complexes bearing no resemblance whatever to the usual QRS complexes are almost surely ventricular, while wide premature QRS complexes whose initial portions are very much like those of the normal beats are probably supraventricular.

If doubt still remains about the origin of the premature beat, an examination of the pause after the premature beat can be very helpful. From it we can determine whether the sinoatrial node has been depolarized and reset by the premature beat. We know that the atria are always depolarized by atrial premature beats, usually depolarized by junctional premature beats and only infrequently depolarized by ventricular premature beats; thus if we find that the sinoatrial pacemaker has been reset, the premature beat is probably supraventricular, while if the sinus rhythm continues undisturbed, the beat is probably a VPB.

Look again at Figure 3-13. The basic rhythm is regular sinus rhythm at 92 per minute, giving a PP interval of .66 second except where there are premature beats. When the PP interval is measured between the two normal beats on either side of a premature beat, it is 1.32 seconds, exactly twice normal. Therefore, even though we can't see a P wave anywhere around the premature QRS complexes, we can infer that there has been no premature atrial depolarization to disturb the regularity of the sinoatrial pacemaker. When the first sinus beat after a premature beat comes right on time, not early, then the pause between the premature beat and the sinus beat is called a *full compensatory pause*.

Figure 3-14 is a rhythm strip showing obvious atrial premature beats. The basic rhythm is sinus bradycardia at 49 per minute, so the normal PP interval is 1.22 seconds. However, the PP interval between the two sinus beats on either side of the first APB is 1.90 seconds, indicating less than a full compensatory pause—the expected finding with supraventricular premature beats.

The arrows in Figure 3-14 demonstrate the resetting of the sinoatrial pacemaker. The dotted arrow shows where a P wave would have appeared after the premature beat had the sinus rhythm continued undisturbed. However, the sinus P wave (open arrow) actually appeared .54 second sooner than expected, proving that the sinus pacemaker had been reset. The new sinus rhythm continued for only

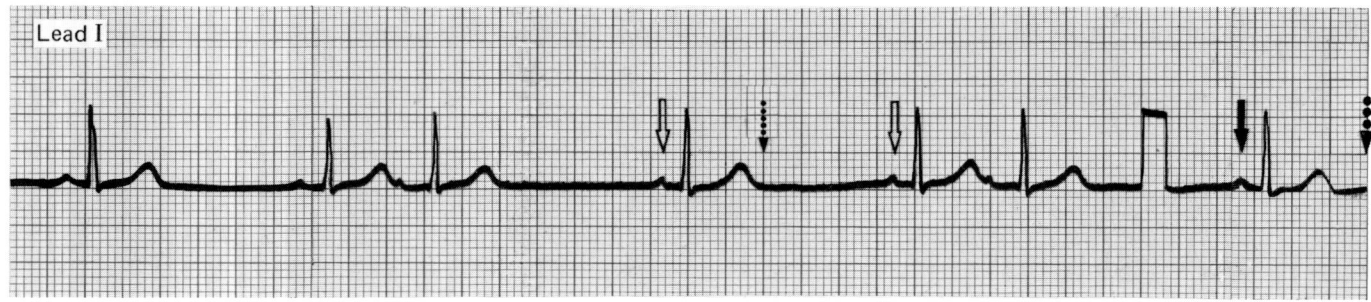

Figure 3-14.

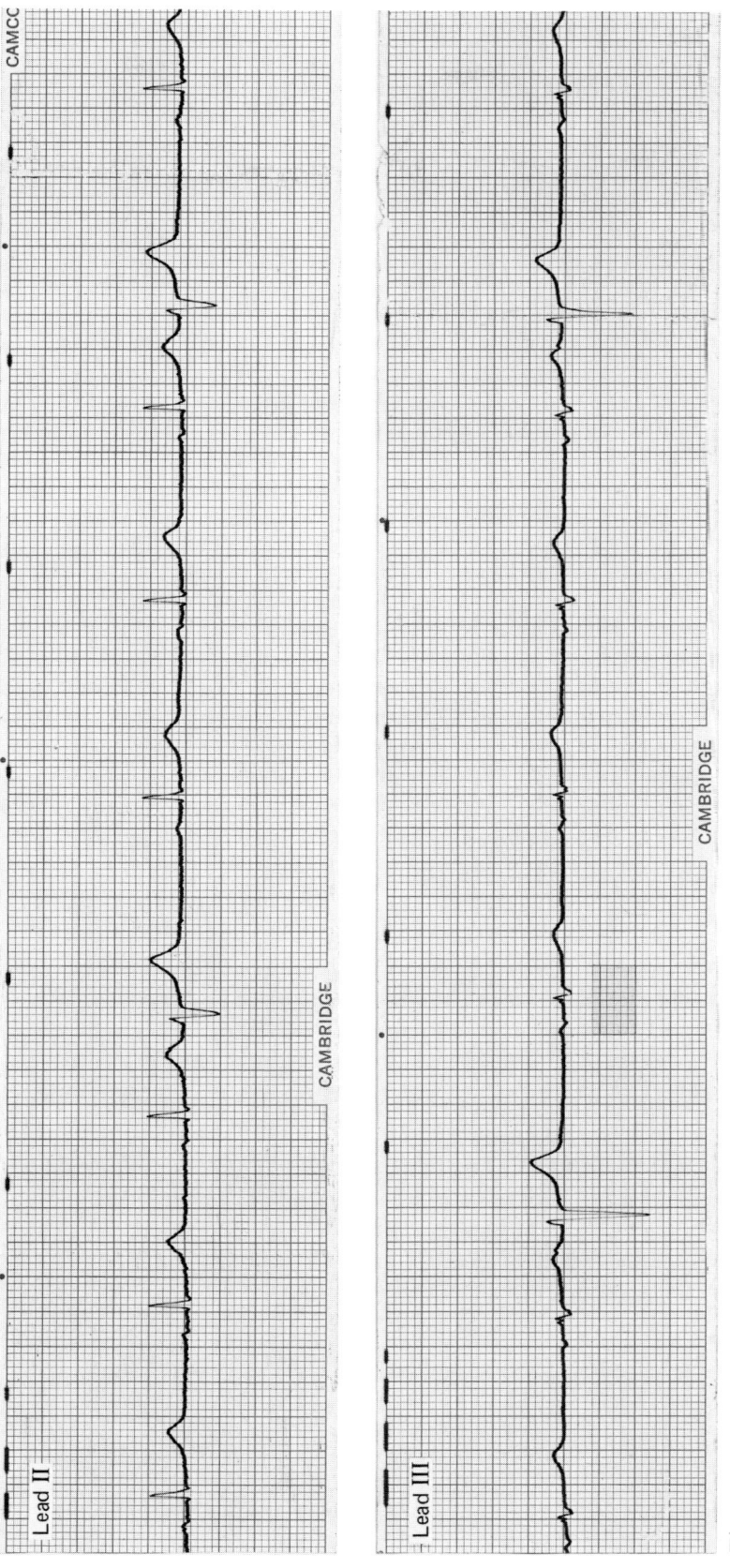

Figure 3-15.

58 / Basic Electrocardiography Handbook

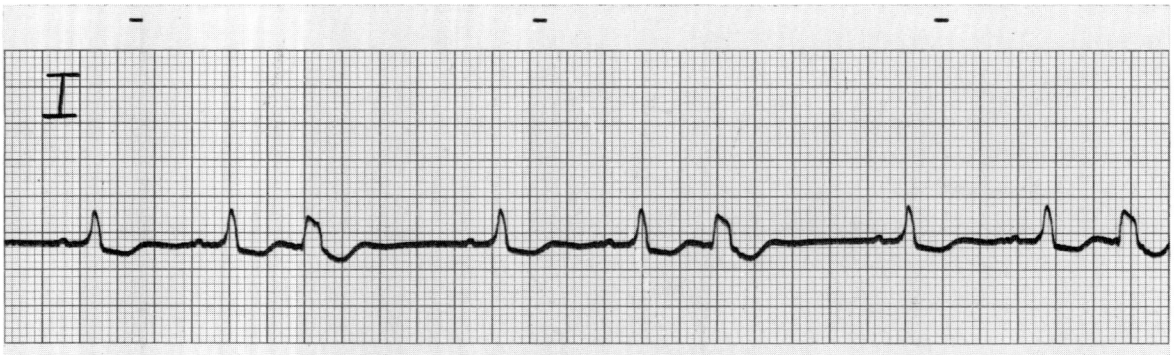

Figure 3-16.

two beats when it was interrupted by an APB. Again the sinoatrial pacemaker was reset; there was less than a full compensatory pause, so the next sinus beat (solid arrow) again appeared earlier than expected (large, dotted arrow).

Figures 3-15, 3-16 and 3-17 are rhythm strips from three different patients. Analyze each one to determine the origin of the premature beats before going on to the explanation that follows.

Figure 3-15, including leads II and III, shows a sinus bradycardia varying from 50 to 54 per minute, not quite enough for it to be a sinus arrhythmia. When the rate varies like this, use the two normal beats before the premature beat in analysis of the compensatory pause. The PP interval of the two normal beats before the first premature beat in lead II is 1.10 seconds, while around the premature beat, it is 1.86 seconds—much less than a full compensatory pause. Although the numbers are not exactly the same, all the other premature beats also have much less than a full compensatory pause. Therefore, despite the different pattern and the longer duration of the premature QRS complexes, they must be supraventricular. Are there any P waves visible? Not in II, but in III there is a prominent notch only on the T waves preceding the premature beats. These are premature P waves, and with a PR interval of at least .16 second, we make a diagnosis of aberrantly conducted atrial premature beats.

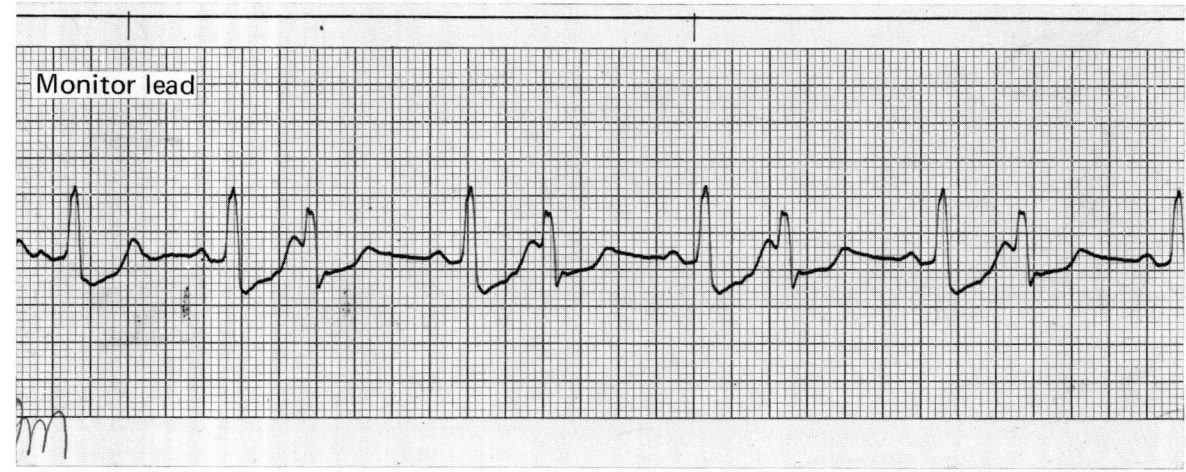

Figure 3-17.

In Figure 3-16, the basic rhythm is a sinus rhythm at 82 per minute, with a PP interval of .72 second. Around the premature beats, the PP interval is 1.44 seconds, a full compensatory pause. There are no premature P waves to be seen, so these are probably ventricular premature beats.

Figure 3-17 is especially tricky, because even the sinus beats have wide QRS complexes. The premature beats have QRS complexes that are similar, but not identical, to those of the sinus beats. Specifically, the premature QRS complexes have a shorter R wave and a definite S wave. The sinus rate is 71, with a PP interval of .84 second. Around the premature beats, the PP interval is 1.25 seconds, much less than a full compensatory pause and strongly suggesting that these are supraventricular premature beats. Are there any P waves? The first ST segment—the only one not followed by a premature beat—ascends in a fairly straight line to the start of the T wave. All the other ST segments contain a notch followed by a small bump just before the T wave and .20 second before the premature QRS, which is very suggestive of a hidden P wave, and provides further evidence that these are supraventricular premature beats, probably atrial.

Now that you have had practice in measuring PP intervals, I should tell you that there is an easier way to determine if a compensatory pause is full or less than full. Take a piece of paper and place it over the electrocardiogram so that the edge is near the baseline but on the opposite side of the main P deflection (Figure 3-18). *Step 1:* Make a short line corresponding to the beginning of the P wave of each of the two sinus beats preceding the premature beat. *Step 2:* Move the paper to the right so the line you made for the first (leftmost) P wave lines up with the second P. *Step 3:* Make another line opposite the first P. Now there are three lines on the paper and the distance from the first to the third is exactly twice the normal PP interval. *Step 4:* Move the paper to the right again so that the newest line is at the beginning of the second P. Look to see where the first P after the premature beat falls with respect to your rightmost line. If the P is just at your line, there is a full compensatory pause. If it is earlier, there is less than a full compensatory pause. Figure 3-18 uses the electrocardiogram from Figure 3-17 to show how the paper should look after each of these steps. Now try it yourself on Figures 3-13, 3-14, 3-15 and 3-16 and any rhythm strips with premature beats that you can obtain where you work.

OTHER SUPRAVENTRICULAR ARRYHTHMIAS

Supraventricular tachycardia is a broad term which includes any supraventricular rhythm faster than 100 per minute. One of the more specific diagnoses listed in Table 3-2 should be made whenever possible, because different treatments are indicated for the various types of supraventricular tachycardia. The key to diagnosis of supraventricular tachycardias is identification of atrial activity. This is usually no problem with the irregular tachycardias, but may prove difficult with the regular ones, particularly if the rate is very rapid.

60 / Basic Electrocardiography Handbook

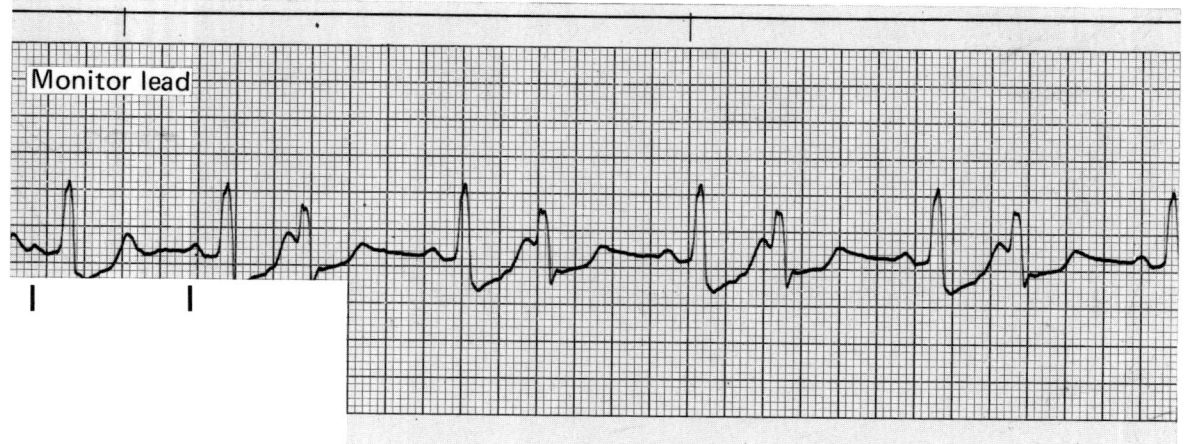

STEP 1

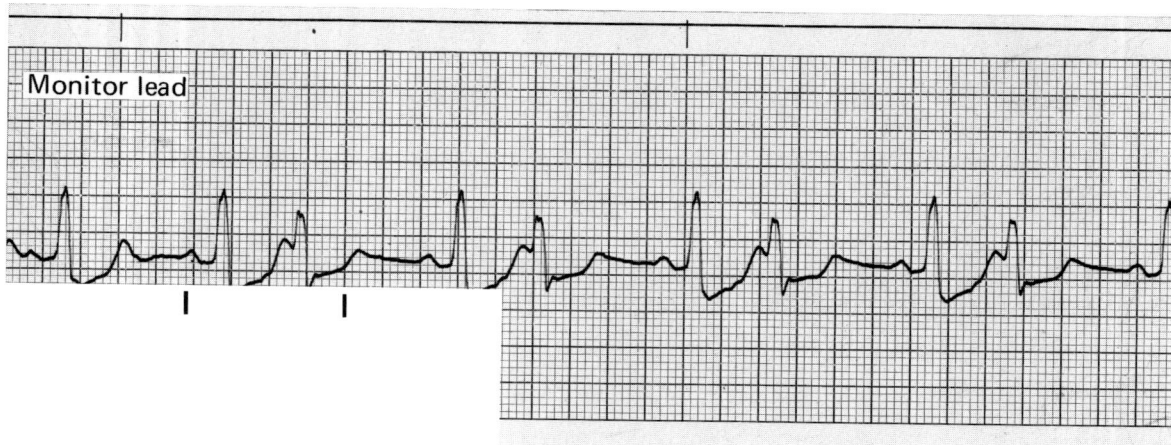

STEP 2

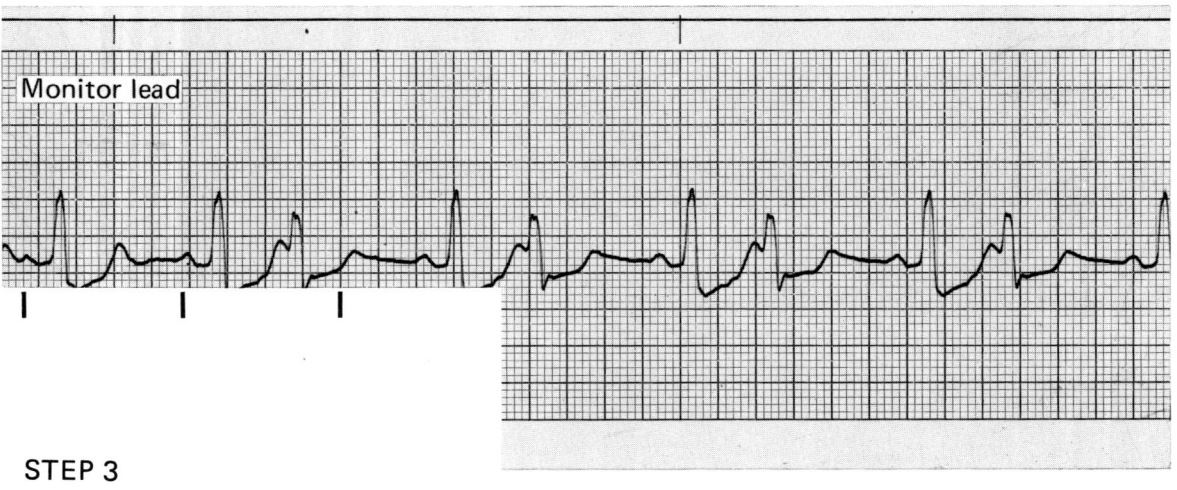

STEP 3

Figure 3-18.

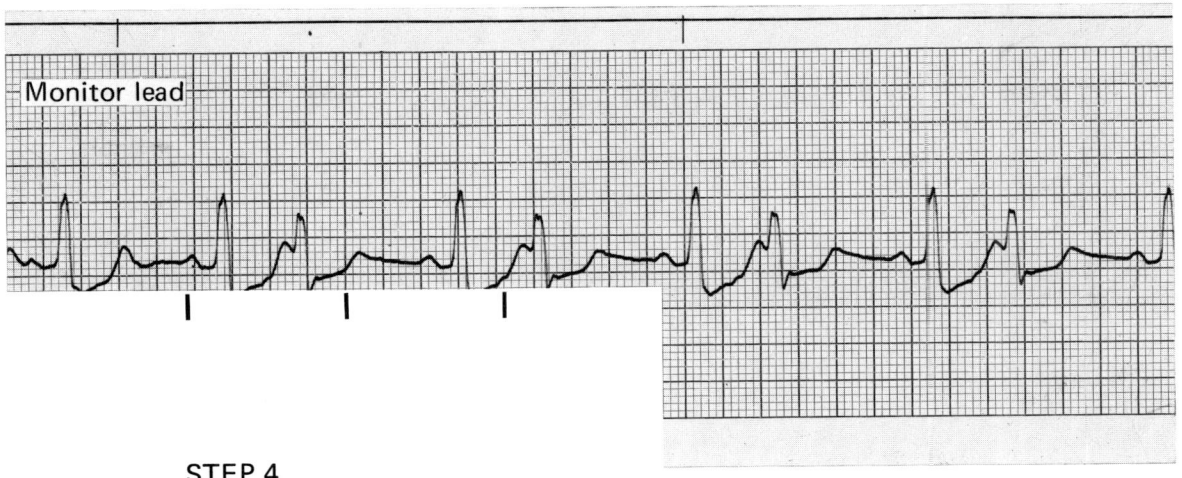

STEP 4

Figure 3-18. (*Continued*).

Only if careful inspection of all leads of the electrocardiogram fails to disclose identifiable atrial activity is a diagnosis of supraventricular tachycardia acceptable.

Atrial tachycardia. Three or more consecutive ectopic atrial beats at a rate of 100 or more are defined as atrial tachycardia. Most cases of atrial tachycardia are paroxysmal with regular, fairly normal-appearing QRS complexes at rates of 160 to 220 beats per minute. Figure 3-19 is a V_1 rhythm strip showing a 19-beat paroxysm of atrial tachycardia at 200 per minute. This example is simple to diagnose because the start of the tachycardia has been recorded and the nearly flat T waves make it easy to identify P waves. Figure 3-19 is exceptional, however. In most cases of paroxysmal atrial tachycardia, such as the one shown in Figure 3-20, the patient arrives complaining of rapid heart-beating, and the electrocardiogram fails to show definite P waves because they are buried in the T waves or the preceding QRS complexes. Under these circumstances, one is forced to diagnose paroxysmal supraventricular tachycardia. Fortunately, at rates close to 200 the only three possibilities in an adult are atrial

Table 3-2. Supraventricular Tachycardia

A. Regular ventricular rhythm
  1. Sinus tachycardia
  2. Atrial tachycardia
  3. AV junctional tachycardia
  4. Reentrant (reciprocal) supraventricular tachycardia
  5. Atrial flutter with fixed block (2:1, 3:1, etc.)
B. Irregular ventricular rhythm
  1. Multifocal atrial tachycardia
  2. Atrial tachycardia with varying block
  3. Atrial flutter with varying block
  4. Atrial fibrillation

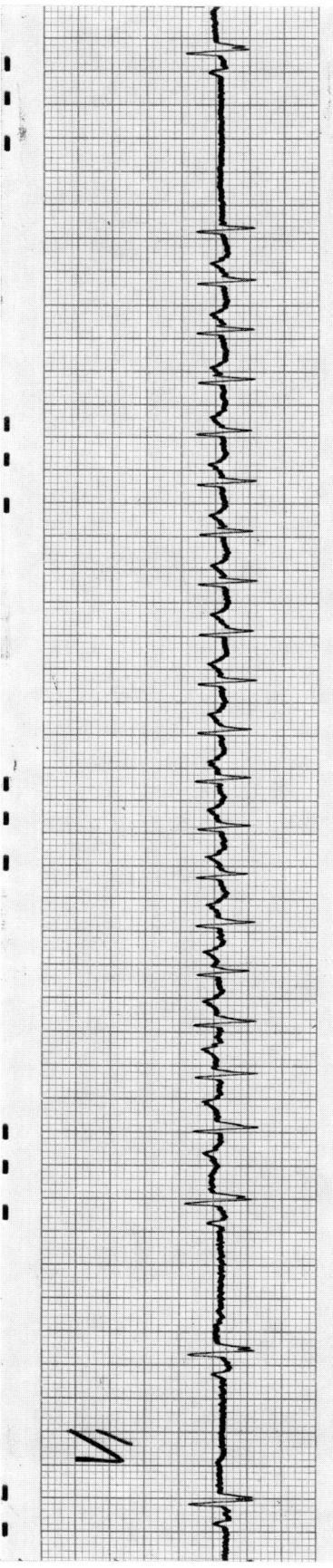

Figure 3-19.

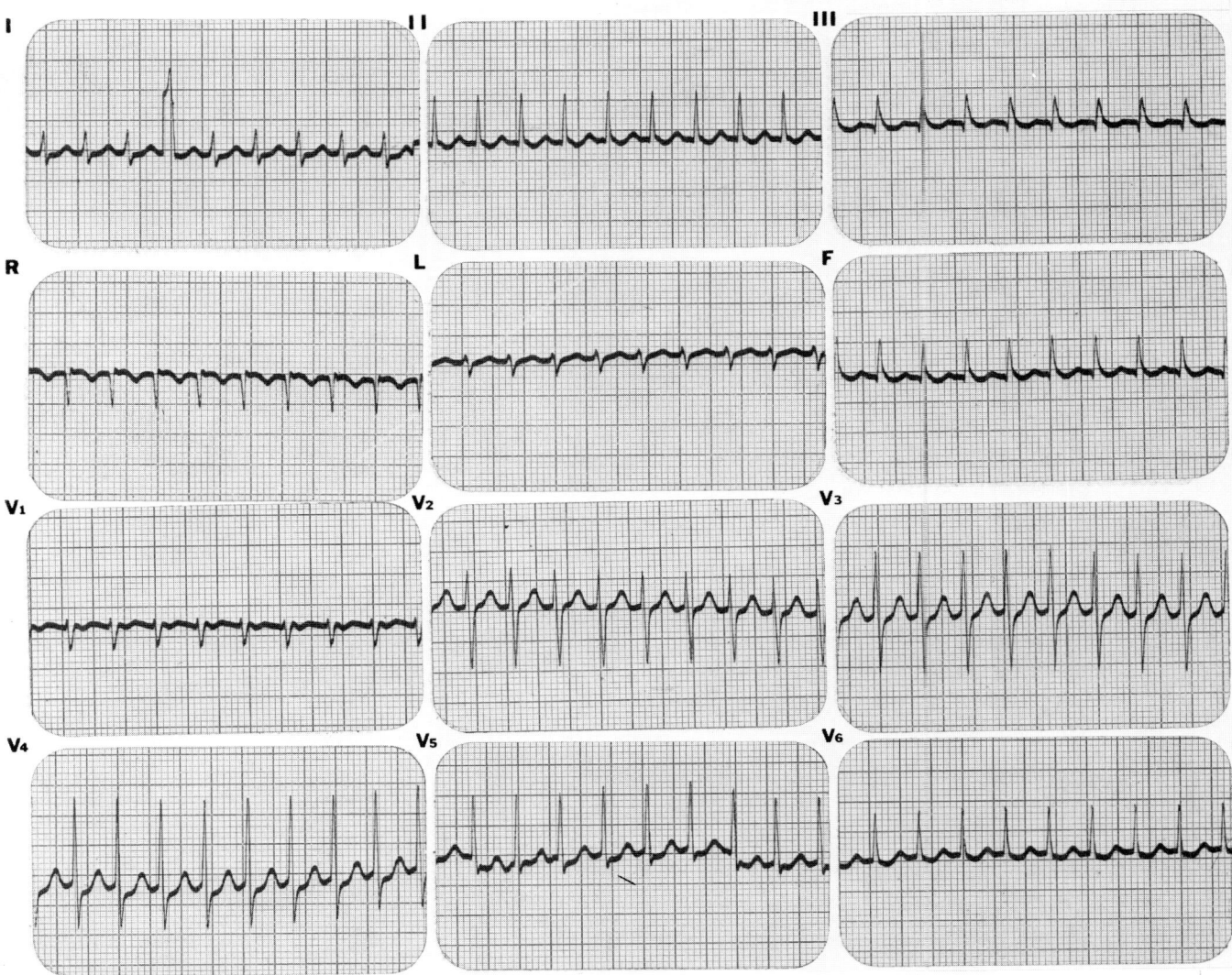

Figure 3-20.

tachycardia, junctional tachycardia and reentrant supraventricular tachycardia, and treatment for all three is pretty much the same.

Usually there is 1:1 conduction in atrial tachycardia, although frequently the PR interval is prolonged. If some P waves are not conducted, the diagnosis is *atrial tachycardia with block*. This diagnosis has special importance because about two-thirds of the cases are caused by digitalis intoxication. Figure 3-21 is a typical example. Regular P waves are present at 175 per minute. In this case, the block varies from 2:1 to 3:2, resulting in a somewhat irregular ventricular response. In a case with a fixed block, there would be a regular ventricular rhythm but at an exact fraction of the atrial rate.

Atrial flutter. In atrial flutter the atria go faster than in atrial tachycardia. The atrial rate is usually around 300 per minute, although it may range from 225 to 350. A diagnosis of atrial flutter should be based on finding typical flutter waves. They usually look like saw

64 / **Basic Electrocardiography Handbook**

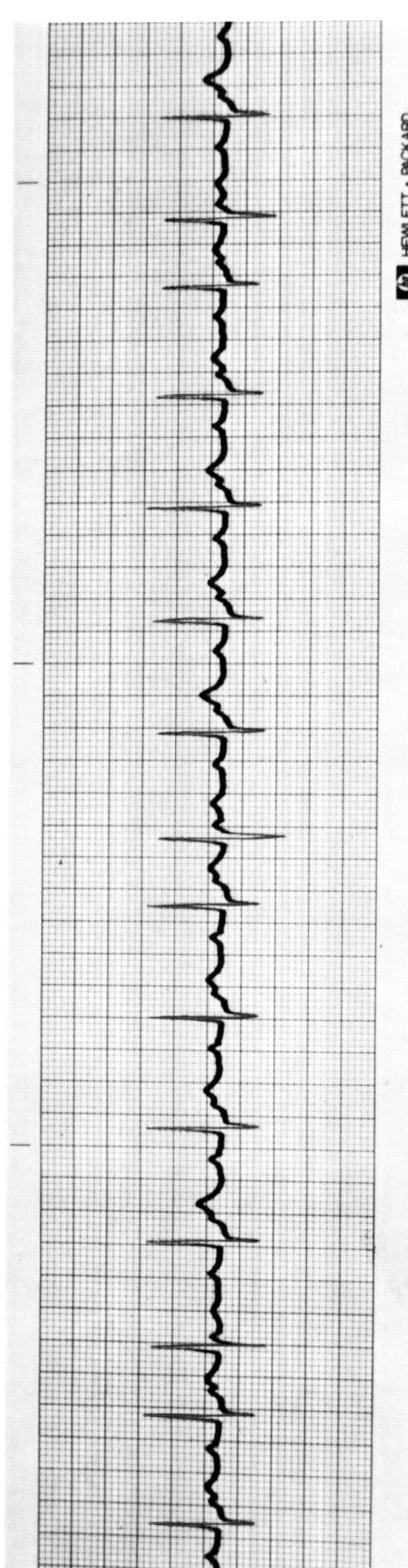

Figure 3-21.

Lead III — Carotid massage

Figure 3-22.

teeth in at least one lead, like those shown in Figure 3-22, a lead III rhythm strip from a case of atrial flutter where *carotid sinus massage* was used to slow the ventricular response and expose the flutter waves. (The carotid sinuses are small structures located on either side of the neck at the branching of the carotid arteries. This maneuver, very useful in the diagnosis and treatment of supraventricular tachycardias, should be performed only by a physician.) The flutter waves are perfectly uniform and regular; however, unlike the P waves of atrial tachycardia, they never return to the baseline, because atrial flutter does not originate from one atrial pacemaker with enhanced automaticity, but rather is caused by an impulse that goes in circus movement around and around the atria, following a fixed path. Each time the impulse comes around to the AV node, it tries to enter it and proceed to the ventricles. But the adult AV node cannot conduct 300 impulses per minute, so atrial flutter is almost always associated with atrioventricular block. With atrial flutter, however, the AV block represents an important safety device, since most ventricles would rapidly fail beating 300 times a minute, and shock or cardiac arrest would follow. The most common form of block is 2:1 block, caused by AV nodal refractoriness to every other beat. In such cases, the ventricular rate is around 150. Since flutter waves are not easy to find among QRS and T waves each occurring 150 times a minute, atrial flutter with 2:1 block is often merely diagnosed as supraventricular tachycardia. However, careful inspection of leads II, III, F and V_1, which generally show the most prominent flutter waves, should indicate the correct diagnosis.

Figure 3-23 is a typical example. First inspection shows a regular, supraventricular tachycardia at 145 per minute without any definite P waves. Because the rate is so close to 150 per minute, atrial flutter with 2:1 block should be strongly considered as a diagnostic possibility. With this in mind, we look again at lead V_1 and are struck by the unusual shape of what appears to be the ST segment and T wave—it seems to slant upward and then drop sharply downward. After that, the baseline slants up again until the next QRS complex. This makes us very suspicious of the presence of flutter waves. However, a conclusive diagnosis would depend on slowing the ventricular rate by drugs or carotid massage. The ventricular rate was slowed in this case; some hours later (Figure 3-24) it was 70 per minute. Now V_1 clearly shows flutter waves at 280 per minute, confirming that the earlier record was indeed atrial flutter with 2:1 block, now slowed to atrial flutter with 4:1 block.

The other common presentation of atrial flutter is *atrial flutter with varying block*. Since there is no fixed conduction ratio, the QRS complexes occur rapidly but irregularly. Again, scrutiny of the baseline should reveal the telltale flutter waves.

Atrial fibrillation is also caused by circus waves, but unlike atrial flutter they follow various paths and frequently collide so that the atria do not really beat, but instead quiver erratically. On the electrocardiogram fibrillatory waves are generally smaller and faster than flutter waves; but the crucial distinction is that, while flutter waves are uniform and regular, fibrillatory waves vary in size, shape

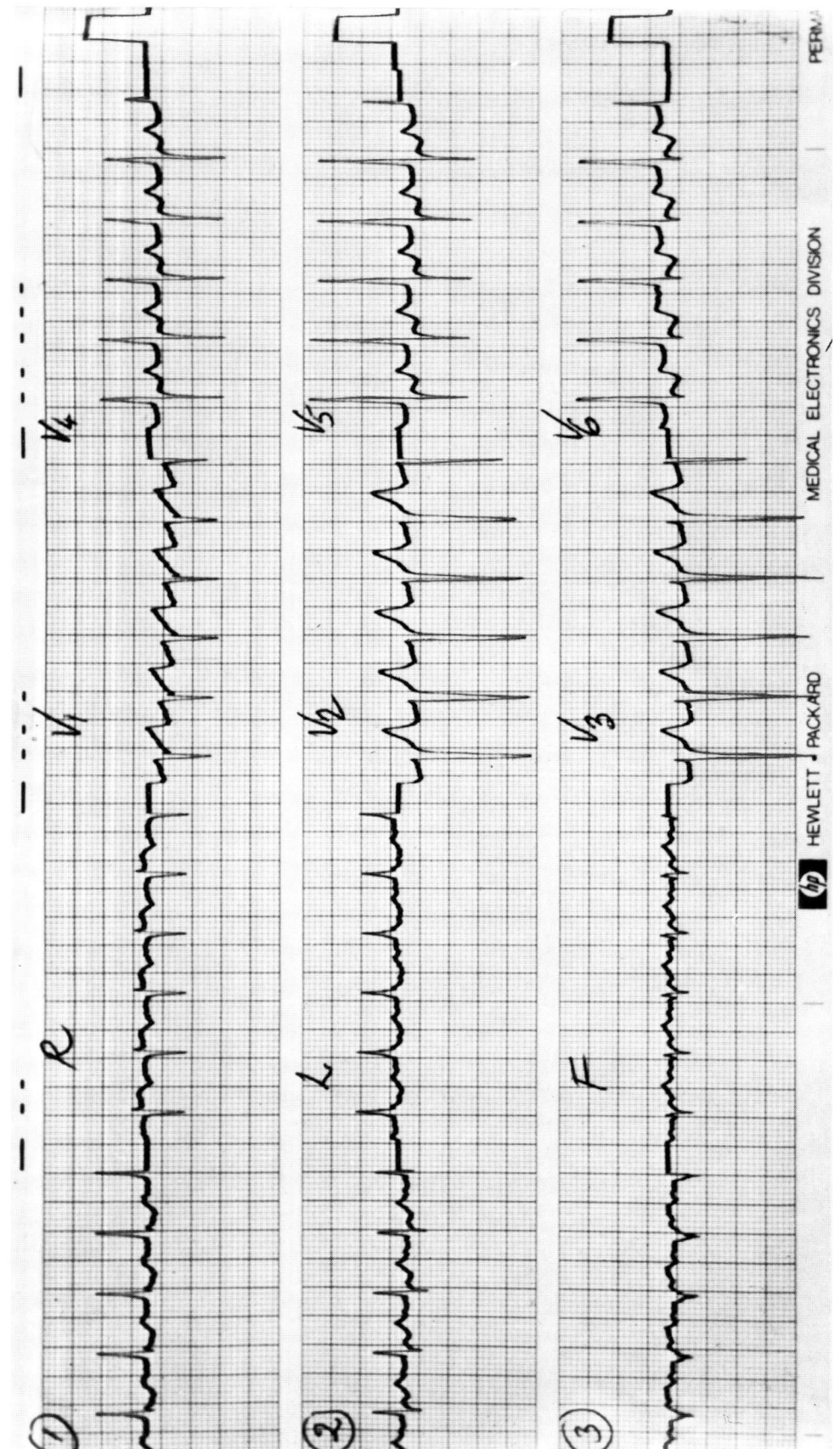

Figure 3-23.

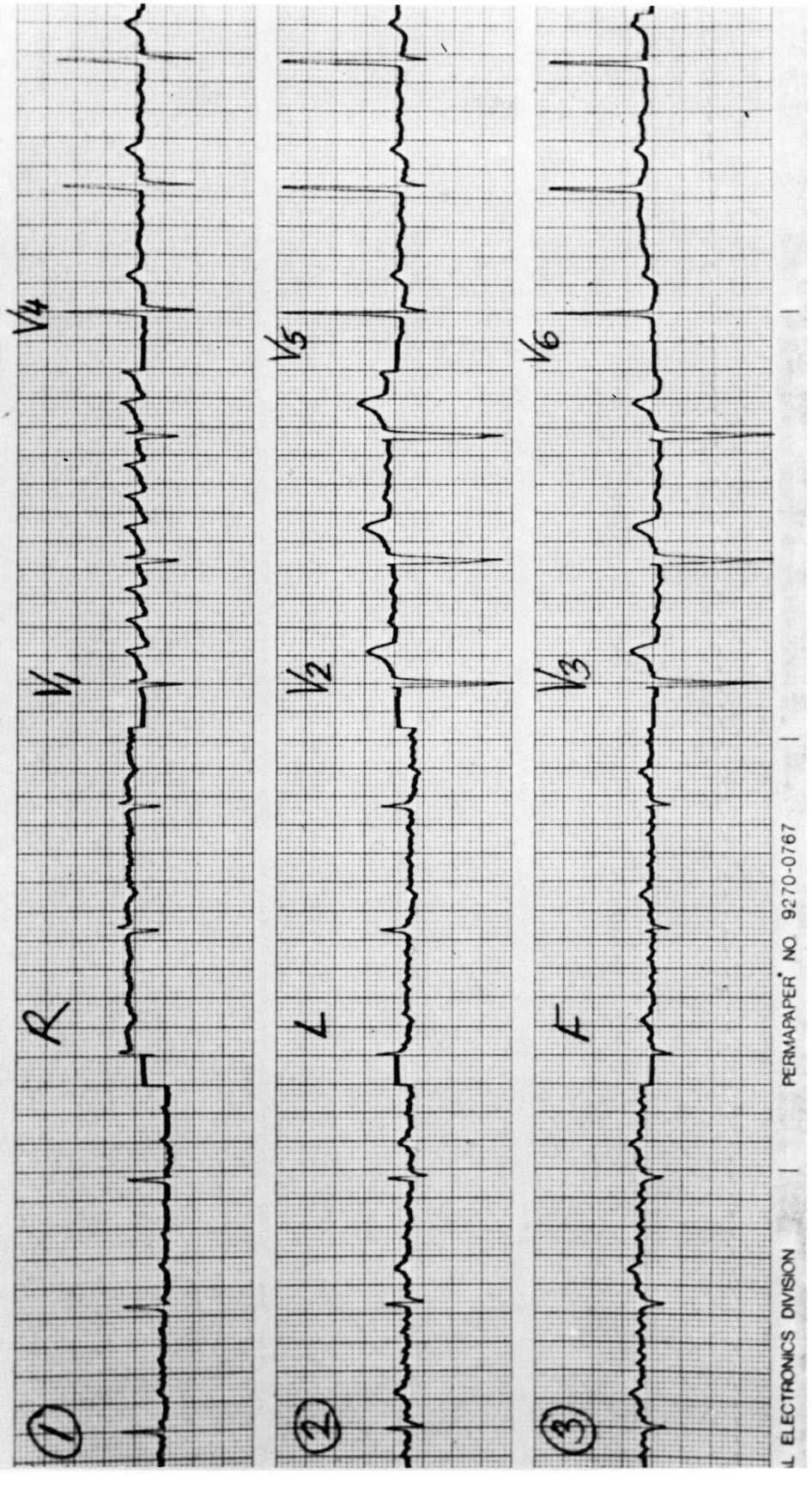

Figure 3-24.

68 / Basic Electrocardiography Handbook

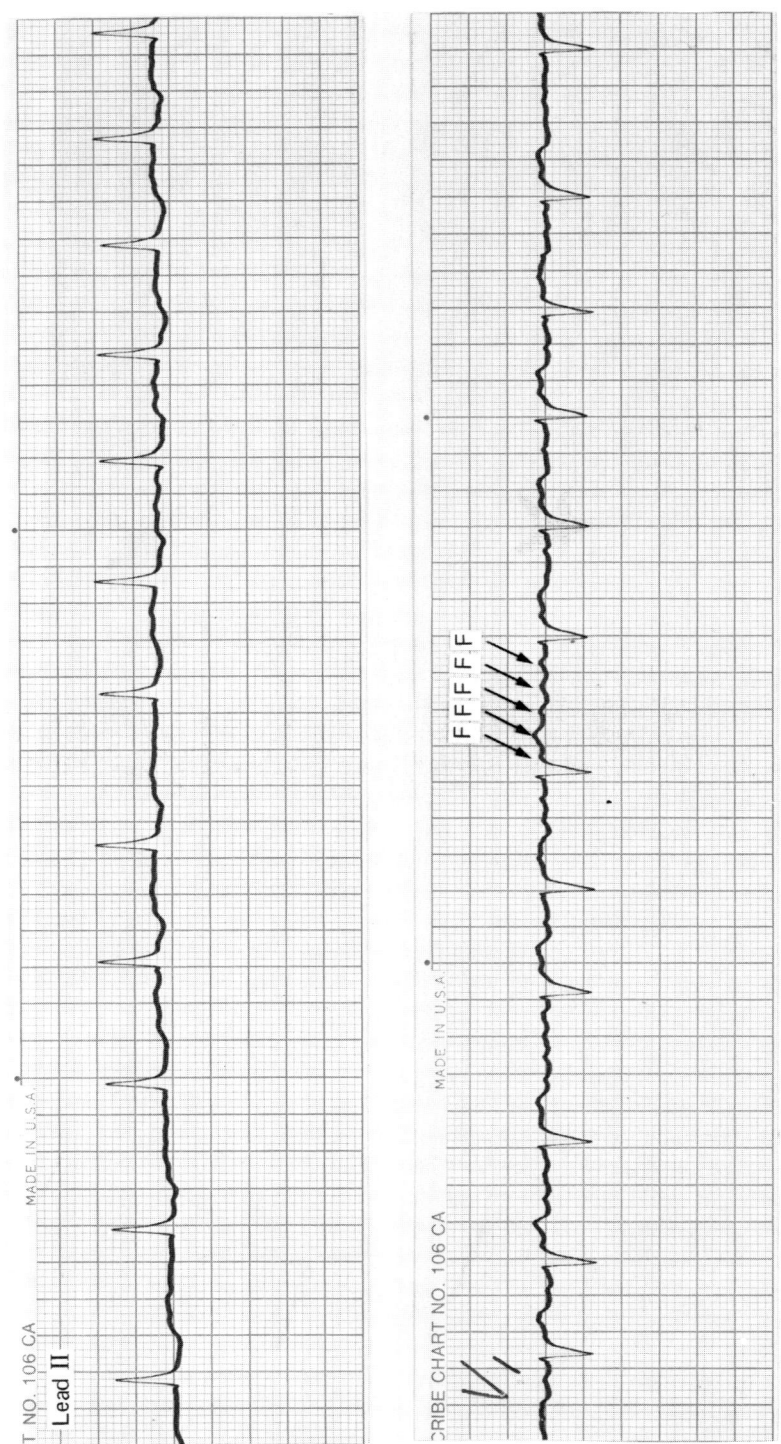

Figure 3-25.

and rate. Sometimes the fibrillatory waves are too small to be seen, or they may be hidden by other waves if the ventricular rate is fast. However, the diagnosis can still be made, because no other rhythm causes complete irregularity of the QRS complexes in the absence of P waves or flutter waves. The usual atrial rate in atrial fibrillation is around 400 per minute. Fortunately, the AV node is refractory to most of these impulses, so the average ventricular rate rarely exceeds 170. The ventricles always beat irregularly in uncomplicated atrial fibrillation—if a regular ventricular rhythm occurs in a patient with atrial fibrillation, then the ventricles are beating independently, so complete heart block or some other form of AV dissociation must be present.

Figure 3-25 shows leads II and V_1 from a patient with typical atrial fibrillation. The fibrillatory waves (F) are obvious in V_1 but barely visible in II. However, the ventricular rate (about 90 per minute) and the rhythm are identical in the two leads, showing the complete irregularity characteristic of atrial fibrillation. Each RR interval is different, ranging from .58 to .84 second.

Figure 3-26 shows lead V_1 from another patient with atrial fibrillation. Because of the rapid heart rate, averaging over 150 per minute, one cannot be certain that fibrillatory waves are present. Nevertheless, the complete irregularity of the QRS complexes plus the absence of well-defined P waves makes the diagnosis of atrial fibrillation. Now you should be able to analyze Figure 3-27.

Lead V_1 of Figure 3-27 shows typical fibrillatory waves. They are also present, but less obvious, in V_6, illustrating again that lead V_1 is one of the best leads for rhythm analysis. However, this tracing is unlike the usual case of atrial fibrillation, because the ventricular rhythm is perfectly regular, at 35 per minute. The atrial rhythm is irregular in atrial fibrillation, so the ventricular rhythm also has to be irregular if the ventricles are responding to atrial impulses. Since this patient has a regular ventricular rhythm, he must have complete AV dissociation; because the rate is so slow, it must be because of third degree block. Therefore, the correction diagnosis in this case is atrial fibrillation with complete, or third degree, AV block.

Aberrant conduction in atrial fibrillation. A difficult diagnostic problem occurs in atrial fibrillation when some beats are much wider than the others. Are the funny-looking beats merely atrial impulses aberrantly conducted, or are they ventricular ectopic beats or runs of ventricular tachycardia? Aberrantly conducted beats are harmless, but ventricular premature beats may indicate a need for different therapy. Unfortunately, there is no completely dependable way to tell them apart, but certain rules are fairly reliable: (1) *Aberrantly conducted beats always conclude a shorter RR interval than the previous one.* Since aberration results from an impulse reaching the His-Purkinje system before all the fascicles have repolarized, the RR interval preceding an aberrant beat must be shorter than the one which precedes the previous normal beat. A longer RR interval preceding the abnormal beat means it must be an ectopic beat. Of course, some VPB's may also conclude short RR intervals; but if the

70 / Basic Electrocardiography Handbook

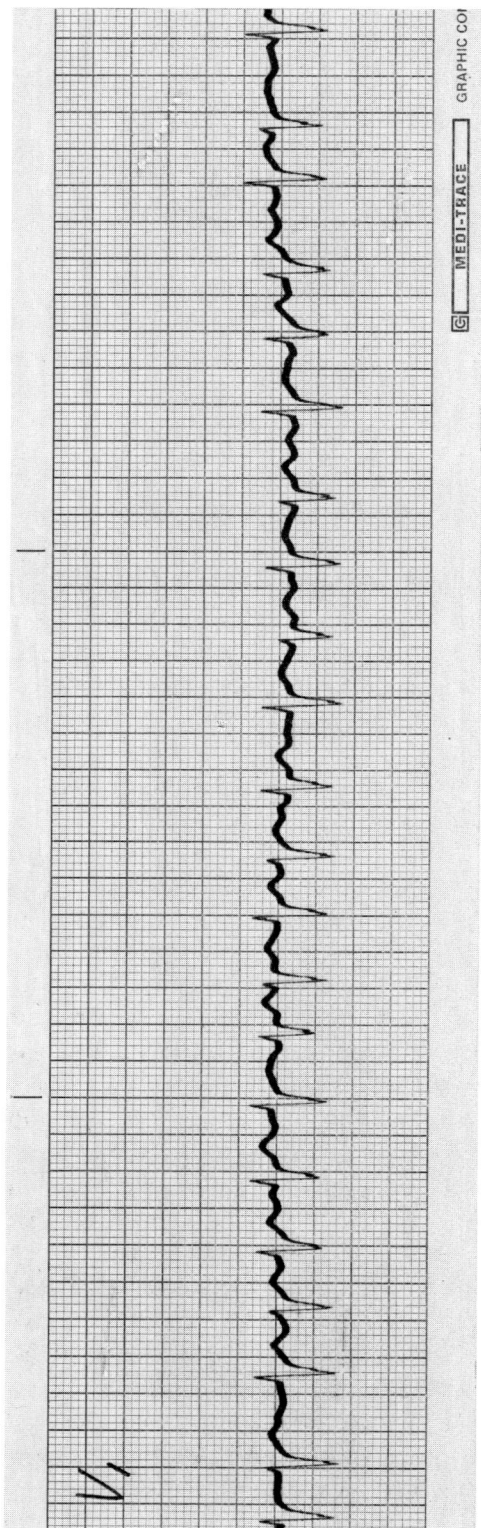

Figure 3-26.

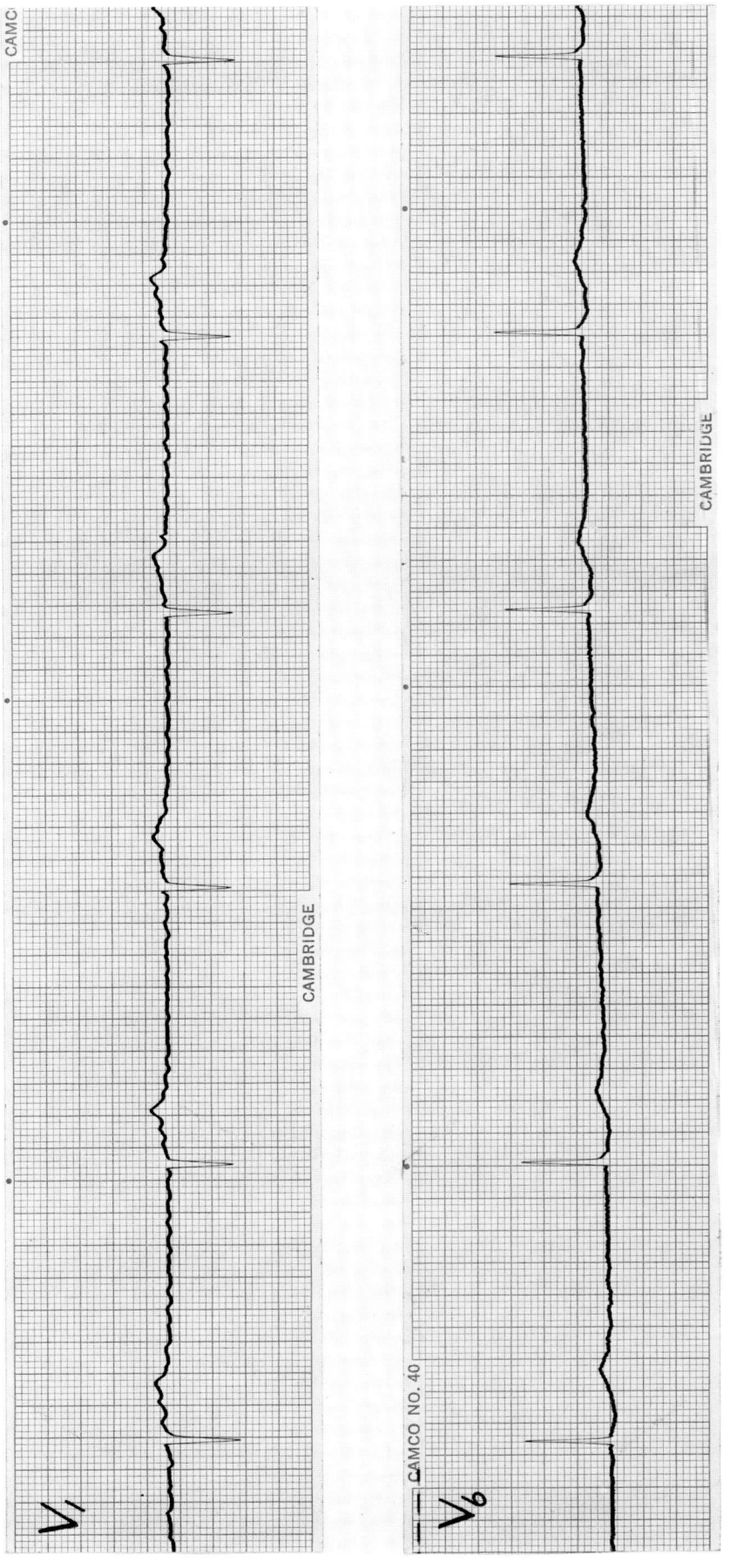

Figure 3-27.

wide QRS complexes are caused by aberrant ventricular conduction, then all of the wide beats will conclude short RR intervals. Again, since aberration results from impulses reaching unrepolarized conducting tissue, the slower the heart rate, the more time the fascicles have to repolarize themselves and the greater the likelihood is that the wide QRS complexes are ventricular ectopic beats; hence, the next rule: (2) *At rapid ventricular rates, aberration is much more likely, while at slow rates the funny-looking beats are probably ventricular.* Two other helpful rules are: (3) *If the RR intervals preceding the wide QRS complexes are all the same, the beats are probably ventricular.* (4) *If every other QRS complex is wide (bigeminal rhythm), they are probably ventricular.*

Sometimes long sequences of beats with wide QRS complexes occur in atrial fibrillation. The same rules apply, plus one more: (5) *If the rhythm of the wide QRS complexes is irregular, and at a rate very close to or identical with that of the atrial fibrillation, diagnose aberration.*

Table 3-3 summarizes the clues that help decide between aberration and ectopy. The more items found from either column, the more likely it is that diagnosis is correct. Apply these principles to the two V_1 rhythm strips illustrated in Figure 3-28. Try to make the diagnosis yourself before reading the next paragraph.

In strip *A*, the average ventricular rate is between 90 and 100; so the rate does not help us in this case. The RR interval from the normal to the wide QRS complex is always shorter than the RR interval before the normal complex. The RR intervals from the normal to the wide complexes are constant, so fixed coupling is present. The rhythm is bigeminal. The wide beats have a QR pattern. In summary, there are three criteria from the ventricular ectopic column and only one

Table 3-3. Analysis of Wide QRS Complexes in Patients with Atrial Fibrillation

Probably supraventricular with aberrant conduction	Probably ventricular ectopic
Atrial fibrillation with rapid ventricular response (over 110/min).	Atrial fibrillation with moderate (60–90) or slow (less than 60) ventricular response.
RR interval from normal to wide QRS complex is *always* shorter than the RR interval before the normal complex.	Some RR intervals from normal to wide QRS complexes are longer than the RR intervals before the normal complexes.
	RR intervals from normal to wide QRS complexes are *always* the same ("fixed coupling").
	Bigeminal rhythm.
Sequences of wide QRS complexes are irregular and at the same rate as the basic rhythm.	Sequences of wide QRS complexes are regular.
RSR′ pattern in V_1	QR pattern in V_1

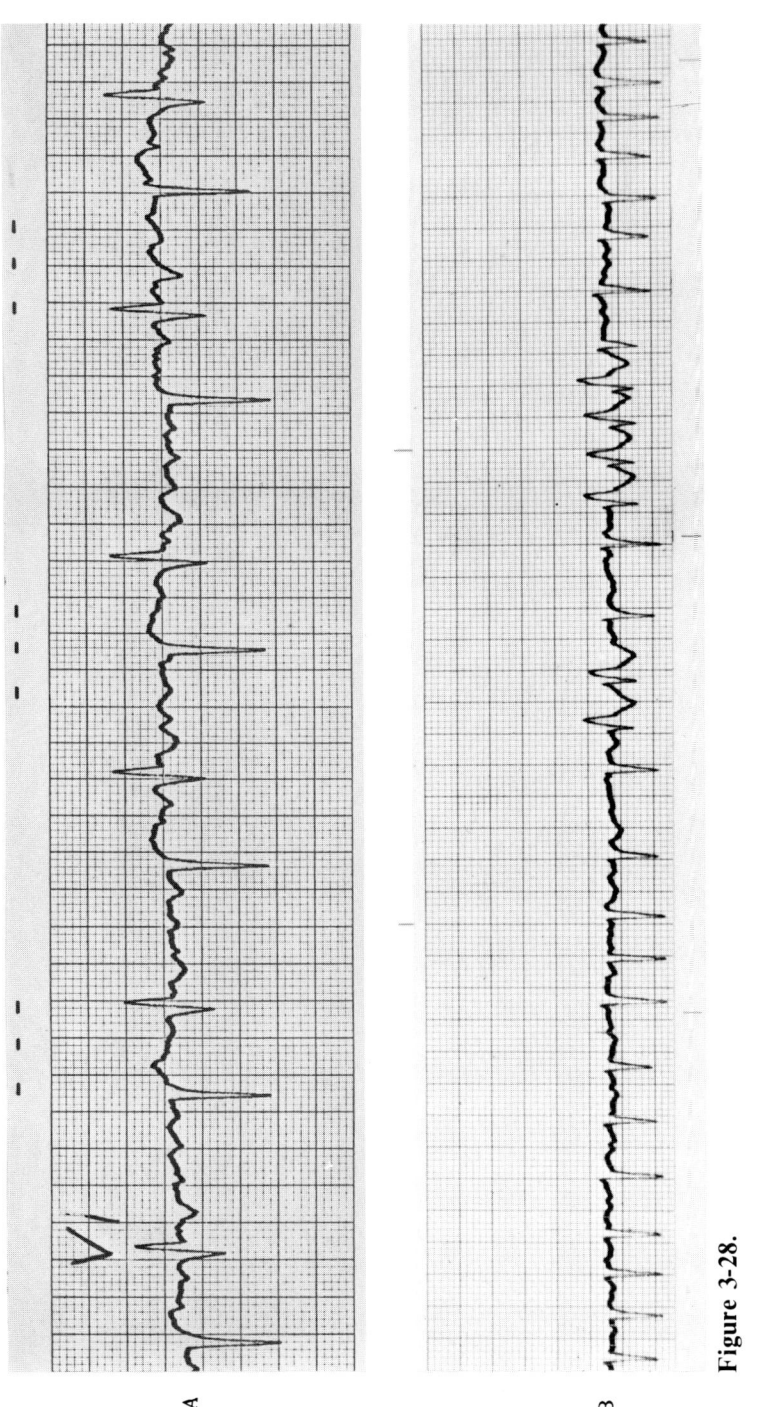

Figure 3-28.

74 / Basic Electrocardiography Handbook

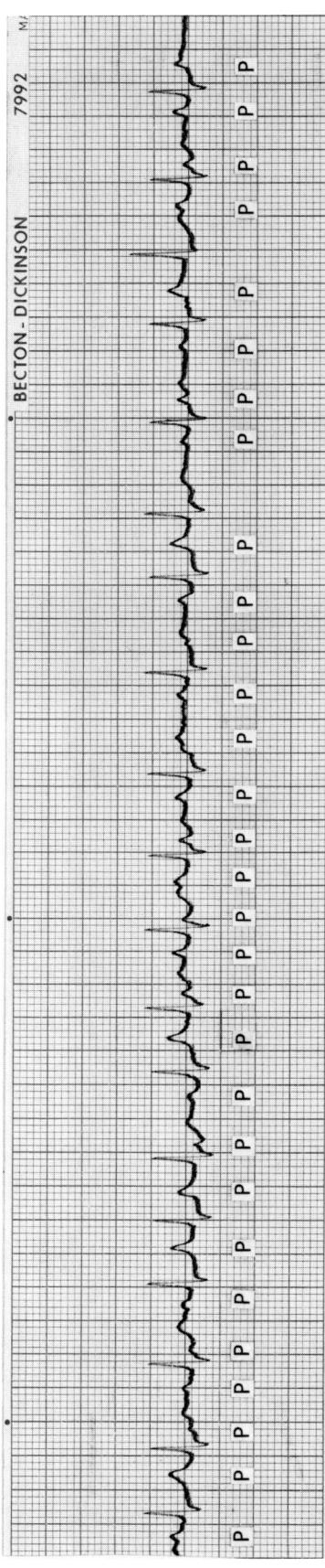

Figure 3-29. (Lead II).

from the aberrant conduction column; so the diagnosis is probable ventricular ectopic beats.

In strip *B*, the basic rhythm is atrial fibrillation with a rapid ventricular response. The RR interval from the normal to the wide QRS complex is always shorter than the RR interval before the normal complex. The sequence of four wide QRS complexes is irregular, and occurs at about the same ventricular rate as the atrial fibrillation. There is an RSR' pattern. In summary, all four criteria for aberrancy are met, and none for ventricular ectopy; so in this case we can make a confident diagnosis of aberrant conduction.

Aberrant conduction is not limited to atrial premature beats and atrial fibrillation, although it seems to be most common in these two arrhythmias. It may be seen with any supraventricular arrhythmia, and the same diagnostic rules apply.

Like atrial fibrillation and atrial flutter with varying block, *multifocal (chaotic) atrial tachycardia* is another cause of a rapid, irregular heart rhythm. Unfortunately, it is often misdiagnosed as atrial fibrillation, which it superficially resembles, but the usual treatments for atrial fibrillation are ineffective and may be harmful in multifocal atrial tachycardia. The tip off is finding three or more distinct P waves in one lead with a straight baseline in between, indicating that the atria are contracting in response to several different atrial pacemakers, rather than circulating waves as in flutter or fibrillation. Figure 3-29 is a typical example. As often happens in multifocal atrial tachycardia, many P waves are not conducted to ventricles.

AV JUNCTIONAL RHYTHMS

Paroxysmal junctional tachycardia behaves very much like paroxysmal atrial tachycardia—it starts and ends suddenly, and the rate is usually between 150 and 200 beats per minute. The diagnosis depends on identification of retrograde P waves, just like those with junctional premature beats. However, the problem of precise diagnosis is the same as with paroxysmal atrial tachycardia, namely that P waves are hard to find at such rapid rates. Figure 3-30 shows a case of paroxysmal junctional tachycardia. The electrocardiogram shows a regular tachycardia at 192 per minute. The narrow QRS complexes indicate a supraventricular origin. There are no clear P waves in any lead. The diagnosis might have been only paroxysmal supraventricular tachycardia, except for Figure 3-31, a lead II rhythm strip taken while one of the patient's carotid sinuses was massaged. The tachycardia was terminated and sinus rhythm promptly returned. However, notice that the final beat of the tachycardia is followed by a retrograde P wave. Furthermore, after three beats of regular sinus rhythm, there is a premature beat with a narrow QRS complex, again followed by a retrograde P wave. Knowing that the last beat of the tachycardia was definitely a junctional beat, and knowing that the patient has junctional premature beats, we can be confident in diagnosing this as a paroxysmal junctional tachycardia.

Accelerated junctional escape rhythm and nonparoxysmal

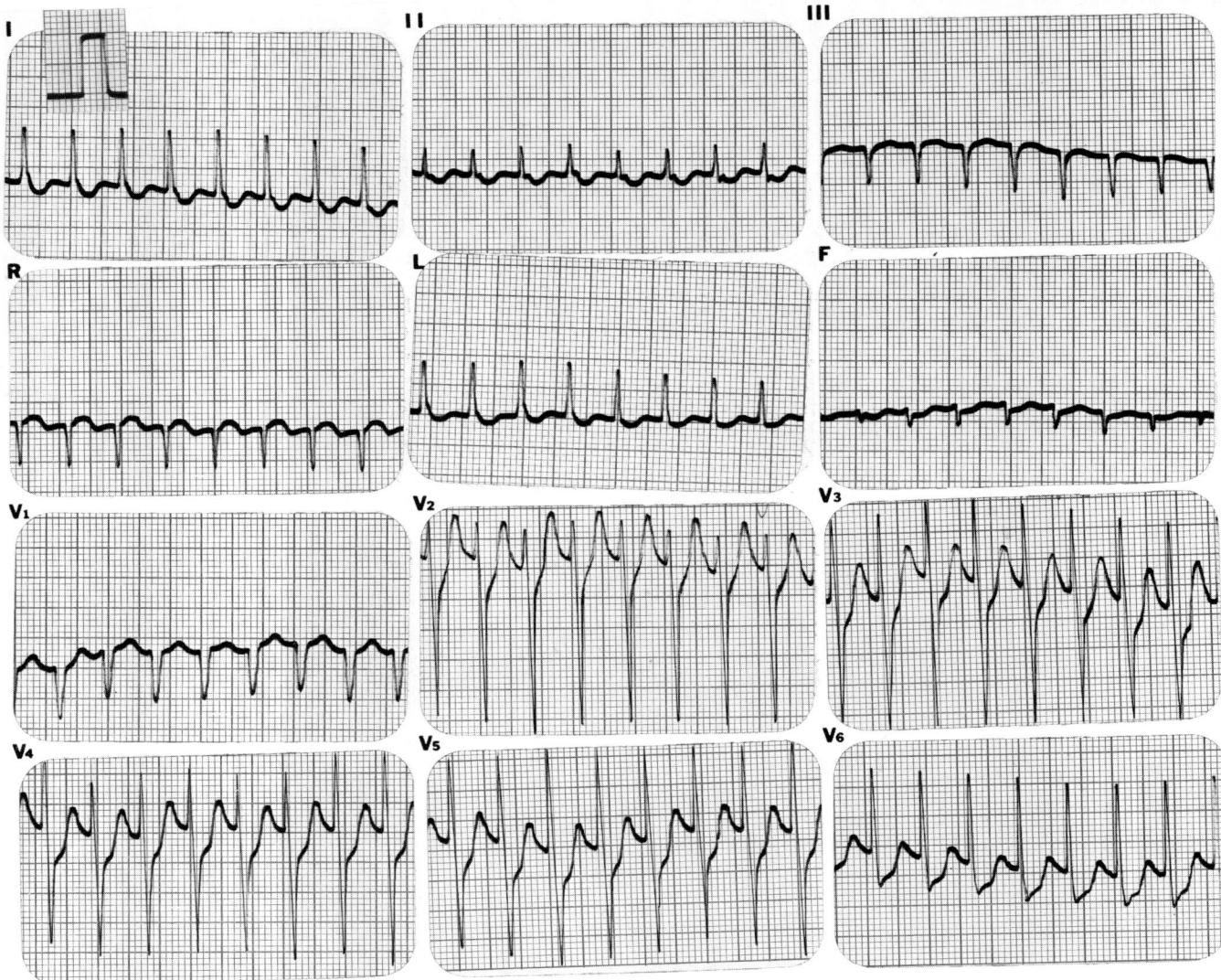

Figure 3-30.

junctional tachycardia have many similar characteristics. Their only difference is the rate. A normal junctional escape rhythm does not exceed 60 beats per minute. Any condition that enhances the automaticity of AV junctional pacemaker cells will cause an increase in the rate of junctional escape rhythms. If the rate is 60 to 70 beats per minute, the diagnosis is accelerated junctional escape rhythm. If the rate is faster than 70 per minute, it is nonparoxysmal junctional tachycardia. Nonparoxysmal junctional tachycardia usually does not exceed 130 per minute, so it is not one of the diagnostic possibilities for a regular supraventricular tachycardia of 150 or more per minute.

Both accelerated junctional escape rhythm and nonparoxysmal junctional tachycardia are nonparoxysmal; that is, they begin by a gradual rate increase, and they end by slowing down over a period of hours to days, not suddenly like a paroxysmal arrhythmia. Both rhythms are caused by the same conditions that depress AV nodal conduction and lead to first degree AV block and type I second degree AV block, namely acute inferior myocardial infarction, digitalis intoxication, myocarditis and recent open heart surgery. There is no

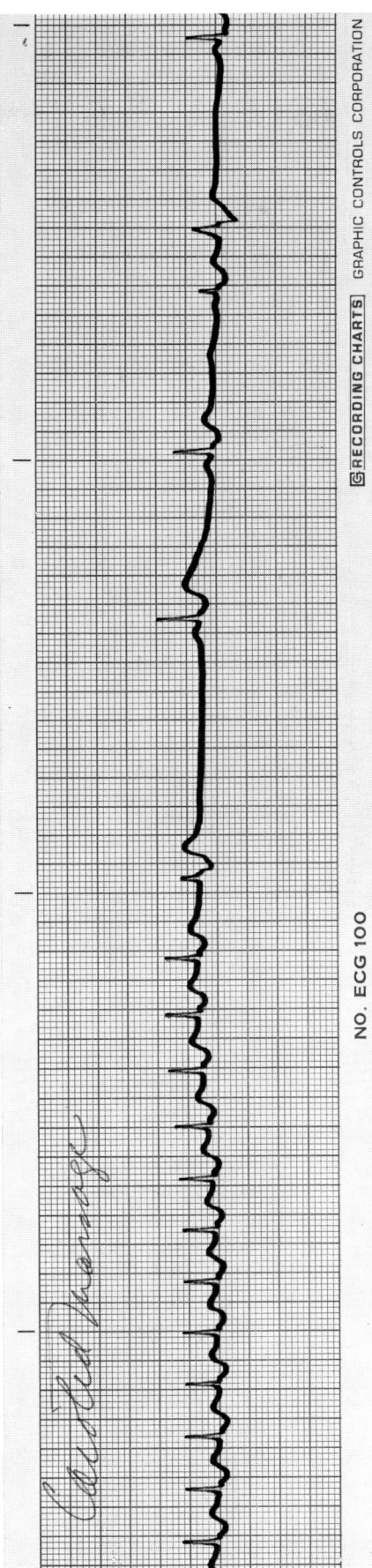

Figure 3-31.

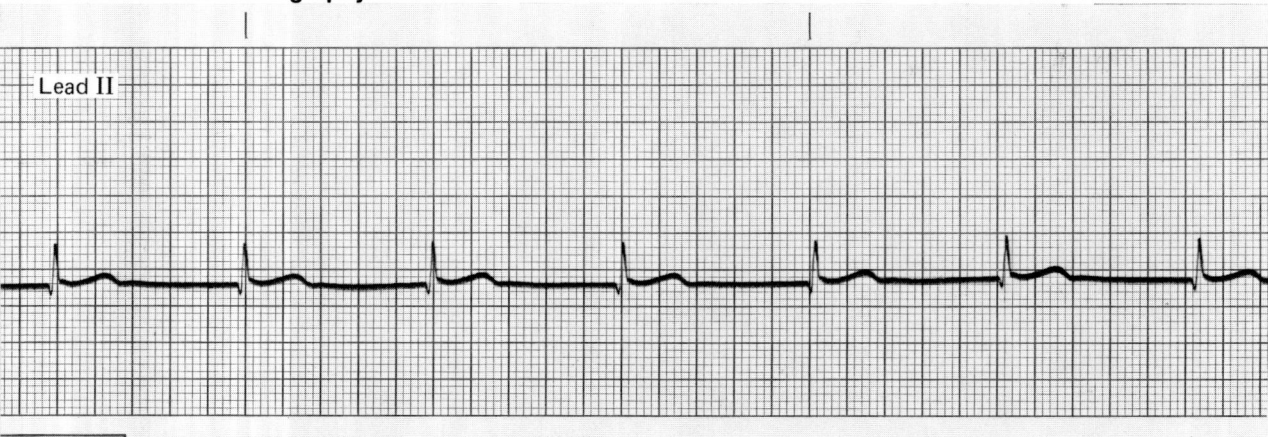

Figure 3-32.

direct treatment for these rhythms. They subside as the underlying condition is treated (digitalis intoxication, some acute myocarditis) or heals with the passage of time (heart surgery, inferior infarction).

Figures 3-32, 3-33 and 3-34 are examples of junctional rhythms chosen to illustrate their properties, and also some of the problems in diagnosis. Try to analyze them yourself before going on to the explanation.

Figure 3-32 is a lead II rhythm strip from a patient with acute inferior myocardial infarction. There are no P waves, but the regular rhythm and the perfectly flat baseline exclude atrial fibrillation; so it must be a junctional rhythm. Since the rate is 59 per minute, it is just called a junctional rhythm. If it were 60, we would call it an accelerated junctional escape rhythm. Since a difference of one beat per minute results in a different diagnosis, is there something crucial about a rate of 60 per minute as compared to 59? No, there isn't, as far as the disease process is concerned. The actual rate of the junctional rhythm depends on how much the underlying disorder— in this case, acute myocardial infarction—enhances the automaticity of the junctional pacemakers. The "magic number" 60, which separates a junctional rhythm from an accelerated junctional escape rhythm, is an arbitrary dividing line, just as is the rate of 70, which separates an accelerated junctional escape rhythm from a nonparoxysmal junctional tachycardia.

Figure 3-33 is a monitor lead rhythm strip from a patient who was overtreated with digitalis. All the QRS complexes look the same, and all are narrow; so we know this is a supraventricular arrhythmia. The first three beats are regular at 100 per minute with no visible P waves, so those beats are a nonparoxysmal junctional tachycardia. Suddenly, a P wave appears after the third QRS complex, and the next QRS complex, marked *C*, comes earlier than expected. (If you are not convinced by "eyeballing" the strip, compare the RR intervals with calipers or, better still, with marks drawn on the edge of a piece of paper.) The early appearance of the QRS complex following a P wave indicates that, at least for that beat, the sinus has captured the ventricles. Such a beat is called a *capture beat*. This particular capture beat begins a run of sinus rhythm, actually sinus arrhythmia because of the rate variations, which continues until the beat marked *E*.

During the period of sinus rhythm, the QRS complexes occur irregularly because of the sinus arrhythmia, and the PR intervals are

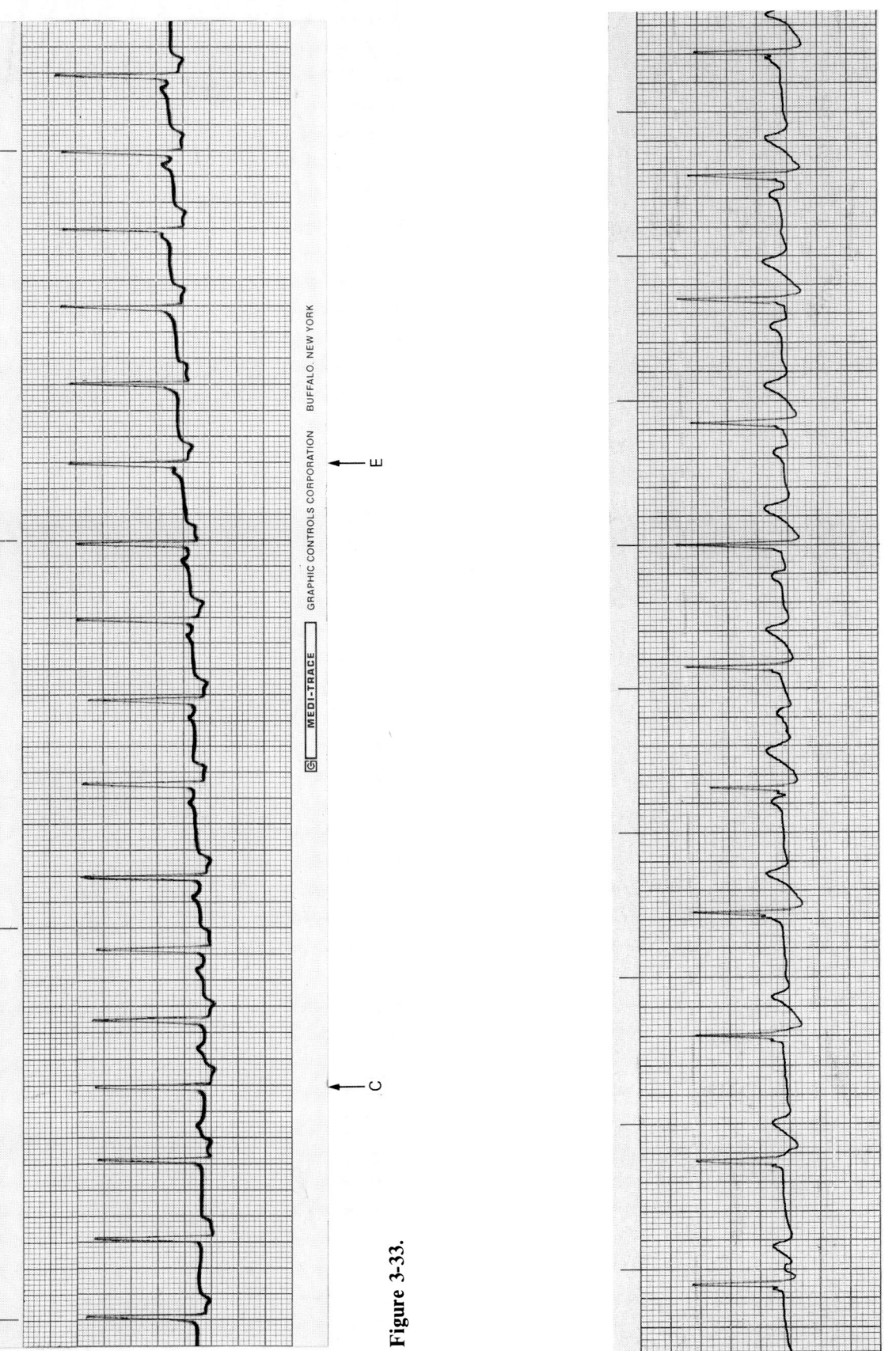

Figure 3-33.

Figure 3-34.

all .16 second. Only the first two PR intervals are longer, but because of increased AV nodal refractoriness, just as with atrial premature beats. Suddenly, at beat *E*, the PR interval shortens to .08 second without any change in the shape of either the P or the QRS. The reason is that slowing of the sinus rate to 90 per minute permits escape of the nonparoxysmal junctional tachycardia, which resumes its previous rate of 100 per minute. For the remainder of the strip, P waves either coincide with, or slightly precede, the QRS complex, but the atria and ventricles are beating independently. We know that because (1) their rates are slightly different, and (2) the atria are slowing down and speeding up while the ventricles continue to beat regularly. Therefore, atrioventricular dissociation is present. Since the AV dissociation is interrupted by periods of sinus rhythm, it is *incomplete AV dissociation*. Even if there were only occasional capture beats, it would still be incomplete AV dissociation.

Figure 3-34 is a monitor lead rhythm strip recorded from another patient with acute inferior infarction. This time P waves are visible except where they are superimposed on the QRS complexes. The sinus rate varies from 80 at the beginning to 100, to 60. Since the P waves are all the same, this is a sinus arrhythmia, not atrial premature beats. Yet, despite the irregularity of the P waves, the QRS complexes (which are obviously supraventricular) are perfectly regular at 71 per minute. Therefore, the ventricles must be beating independently of the atria; so this is also an example of AV dissociation. It is important not to diagnose this as complete heart block even though complete AV dissociation is present and the atria are beating faster than the ventricles, because the escaping pacemaker is an accelerated one, in this case, a nonparoxysmal junctional tachycardia.

A reasonable question at this point would be, "Since the atria are going faster than the ventricles, what allows the junctional beats to escape, inasmuch as the fastest pacemaker is supposed to be the one that controls the heart?" The answer is that some AV block is present. We cannot define it as first degree or second degree, because the rapid junctional rhythm reduces the opportunity for the atria to capture the ventricles. For example, the sixth QRS complex is preceded by a P wave with a PR interval of .32 second, yet the regularity of the nonparoxysmal junctional tachycardia remains undisturbed, showing absence of ventricular capture by that P wave. Therefore, at least first degree AV block must be present. How about second degree? We can't say—perhaps if the P wave came a little bit earlier, ventricular capture would have taken place. In other words, one should not diagnose second degree AV block unless there is failure of some P waves to be conducted to the ventricles at a time when they have full opportunity to do so. Therefore, the answer to the question is that some degree of AV block is present, at least first degree, maybe more, but enough to protect the junctional pacemaker from sinoatrial impulses and permit complete AV dissociation to take place.

TACHYCARDIA-BRADYCARDIA SYNDROME

When a supraventricular tachycardia stops in a patient with a normal sinoatrial node, sinus beats appear almost immediately.

Diagnosis of Cardiac Rhythms / 81

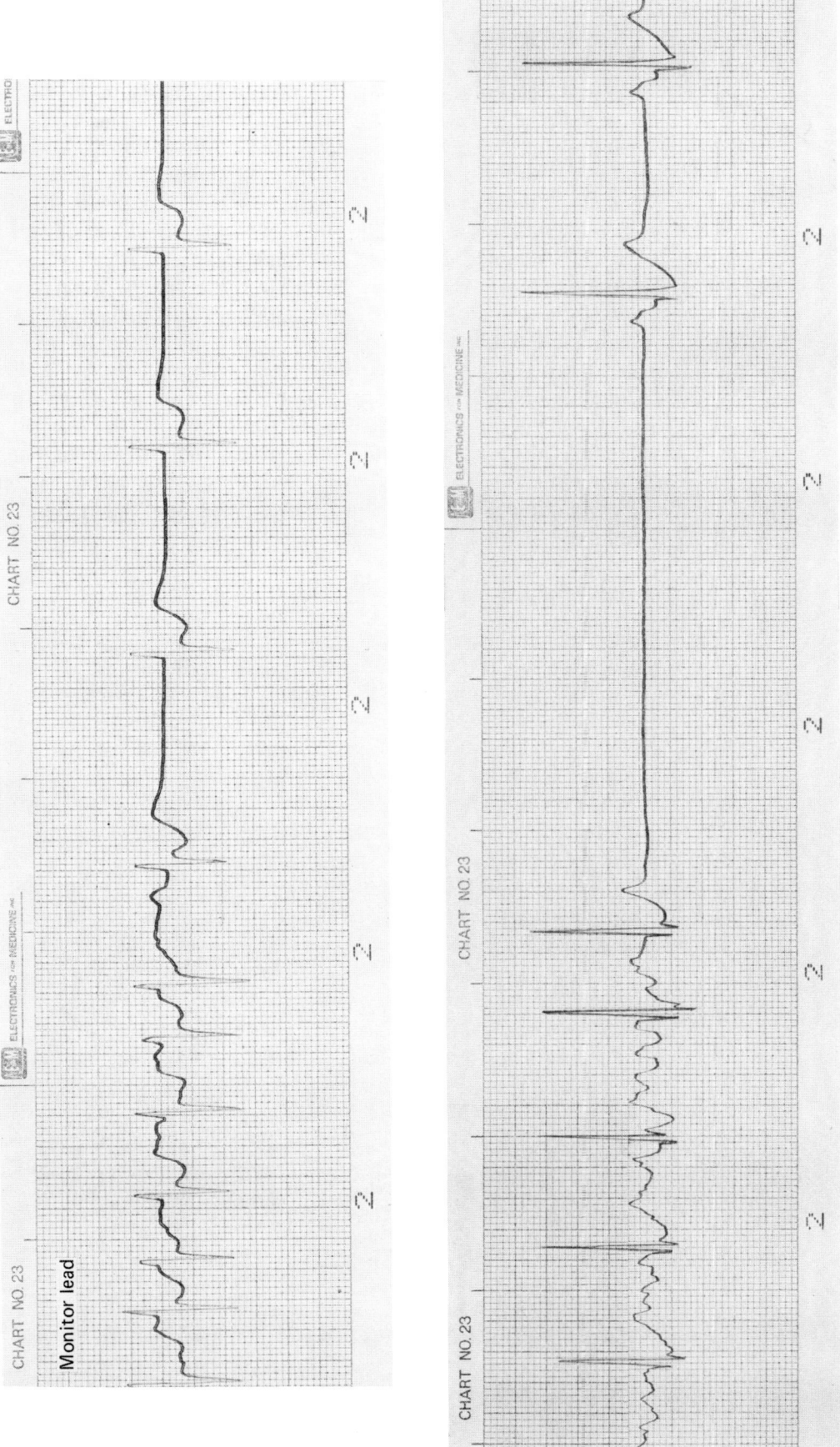

Figure 3-35.

Within a few seconds, a stable sinus rhythm is established and the patient feels better. However, in a patient with a diseased sinoatrial node, sinus rhythm does not immediately recur; instead there is prolonged asystole, severe sinus bradycardia or an escape rhythm. This combination of alternating fast and slow rhythms is called the *tachycardia-bradycardia syndrome*. During the tachycardia, the patients often complain of rapid heart beat; but when the rhythm abruptly slows, they may feel faint or even lose consciousness. Figure 3-35 shows two examples from the same patient, both monitor lead rhythm strips. In *A*, at the end of a paroxysm of atrial fibrillation there is a solitary sinus beat followed by sinus arrest and an AV junctional escape rhythm at 43 per minute. In *B*, a paroxysm of atrial fibrillation is followed by 4 seconds of asystole and then a sinus bradycardia of 40 per minute.

Treatment of the tachycardia-bradycardia syndrome is difficult if drugs alone are used, because the drugs that are useful for preventing or slowing tachycardia frequently make the bradycardias worse, and drugs to speed up the bradycardia often increase the rate and the frequency of tachycardias. As a result, many patients require a combination of treatment with drugs for the tachycardia and a pacemaker to eliminate the bradycardia.

VENTRICULAR ARRHYTHMIAS

Accelerated idioventricular rhythm is a regular, ventricular rhythm between 45 and 100 beats per minute. It usually appears as an escape rhythm at times when the sinoatrial pacemaker slows, particularly when the patient is asleep. Because the rate of accelerated idioventricular rhythm is close to that of sinus rhythm, it usually begins and ends with fusion beats (see below). Furthermore, accelerated idioventricular rhythm rarely lasts for more than 30 beats; so there is usually no major effect on cardiac output and no need for the kind of urgent treatment indicated for the faster and more dangerous ventricular arrhythmias. Since accelerated idioventricular rhythm most often occurs in patients with acute myocardial infarction, the very patients who usually receive the most vigorous treatment for other ventricular arrhythmias, the diagnosis of accelerated idioventricular rhythm is an especially important one to make so that the patient will not receive unnecessary therapy.

Figure 3-36 is a monitor lead rhythm strip recorded from a patient with an acute myocardial infarction. The first and last beats are sinoatrial beats to show the patient's usual QRS complexes. Beats 2 through 10 are an accelerated idioventricular rhythm at 64 per minute. Beats 3 through 9 have the expected appearance of ventricular beats—they are wide and obviously different from the patient's normal QRS complexes. But beats 2 and 10 don't really look like ventricular beats; they don't look like the sinus beats, either—in fact, they have QRS configurations intermediate between those of the ventricular and the sinus beats. Furthermore, these beats are preceded by P waves, but the PR interval is shorter than the patient's usual PR interval of .16 second. These two beats are *fusion beats*, that is, they

Diagnosis of Cardiac Rhythms / 83

Figure 3-36.

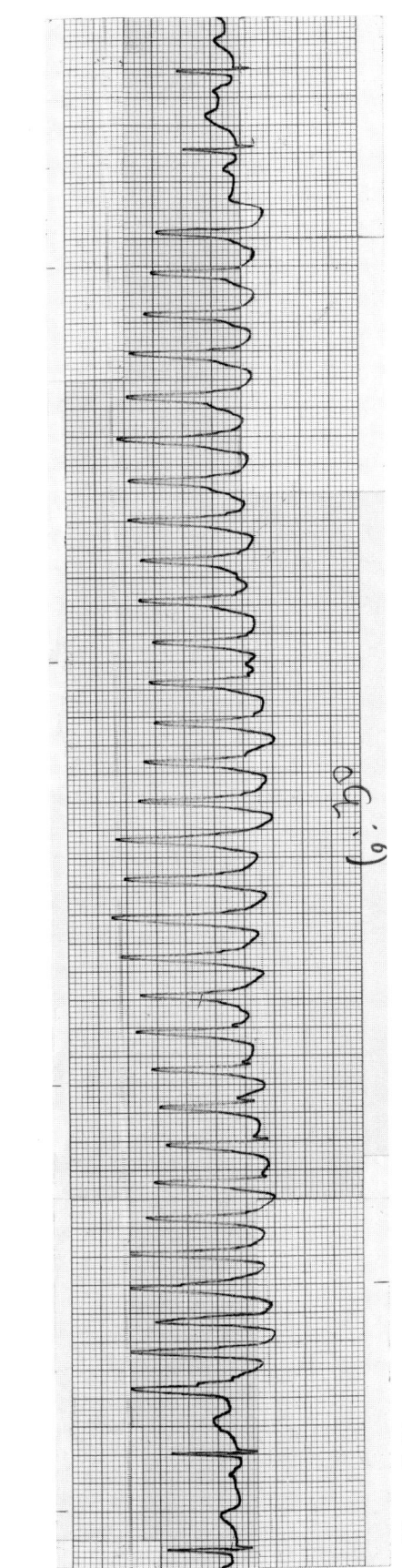

Figure 3-37.

are the result of ventricular depolarization by two different pacemakers—in this case, the sinoatrial node and the ectopic ventricular pacemaker. Fusion beats are often a helpful diagnostic clue in rhythm analysis, because they are proof that two independent pacemakers are functioning in the heart. (The only exception to this rule is Wolff-Parkinson-White syndrome, in which one impulse reaches the ventricle by two pathways, and so has the same effect as two independent pacemakers.) Depending on whether more of the ventricle is depolarized by the sinoatrial or the ectopic pacemaker, the fusion beat will look more like either a sinoatrial beat (beat 2) or a ventricular beat (beat 10).

Ventricular tachycardia is a regular, or slightly irregular, ventricular rhythm whose rate may be anywhere from 100 to 300 beats per minute. Particularly at faster rates, ventricular tachycardia results in a marked reduction in cardiac output; so patients may develop low blood pressure or *syncope* (fainting) or go into shock. Urgent treatment is often required. The QRS configuration may remain the same or change during the tachycardia, but after the initial warmup period the rate is relatively constant. The main problems in diagnosis are differentiating ventricular tachycardia from (1) a regular supraventricular tachycardia with bundle branch block or aberrant conduction and (2) atrial fibrillation with bundle branch block or aberrant conduction.

Figure 3-37 is a monitor lead rhythm strip showing an 8-second paroxysm of ventricular tachycardia. If you are fortunate enough to be able to record or have monitoring equipment sophisticated enough to recall the first beat of any type of tachycardia, the diagnosis should be easy to make. In this case two normal-appearing sinus beats are followed by an obvious ventricular premature beat which initiates the tachycardia. There is some irregularity of the first few beats; then the tachycardia settles down to a steady 210 beats per minute until it ends.

If only the last 3 or 4 seconds of the tachycardia had been recorded, it would be more difficult to be sure this was a ventricular tachycardia without additional evidence, such as that provided by Figure 3-38, another rhythm strip from the same patient (please pardon the respiratory artefact). Every fourth beat is a ventricular premature beat, and these VPB's look just like the QRS complexes of the tachycardia. As a rule, it is easier to identify the origin of a single premature beat than an established tachycardia. If there are premature beats whose QRS complexes are identical to or strongly resemble those of the tachycardia, that is good evidence that the tachycardia arises from the same part of the heart as the premature beats.

Seeing the start of the tachycardia or finding premature beats that look like the tachycardia are probably the two most reliable ways to differentiate ventricular from supraventricular tachycardias. However, there are other useful clues, some of which are illustrated by Figure 3-39 which shows a regular tachycardia at 155 per minute with wide QRS complexes. Is it ventricular or supraventricular?

The QRS pattern in V_1 is QR—this favors ventricular tachycardia just as an RSR' would favor a supraventricular tachycardia (see Table 3-3). Capture beats, that is, early QRS complexes that appear less

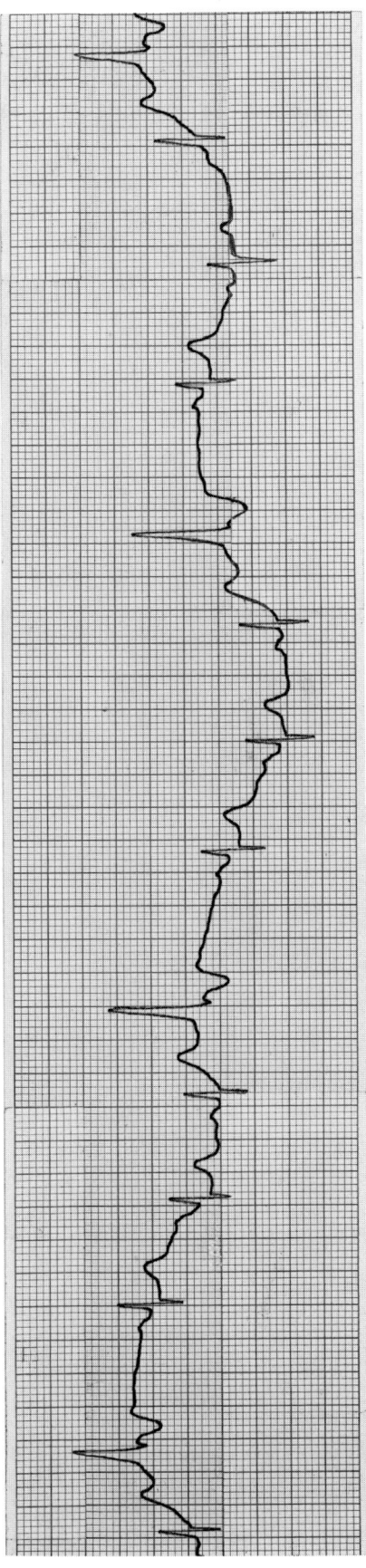

Figure 3-38.

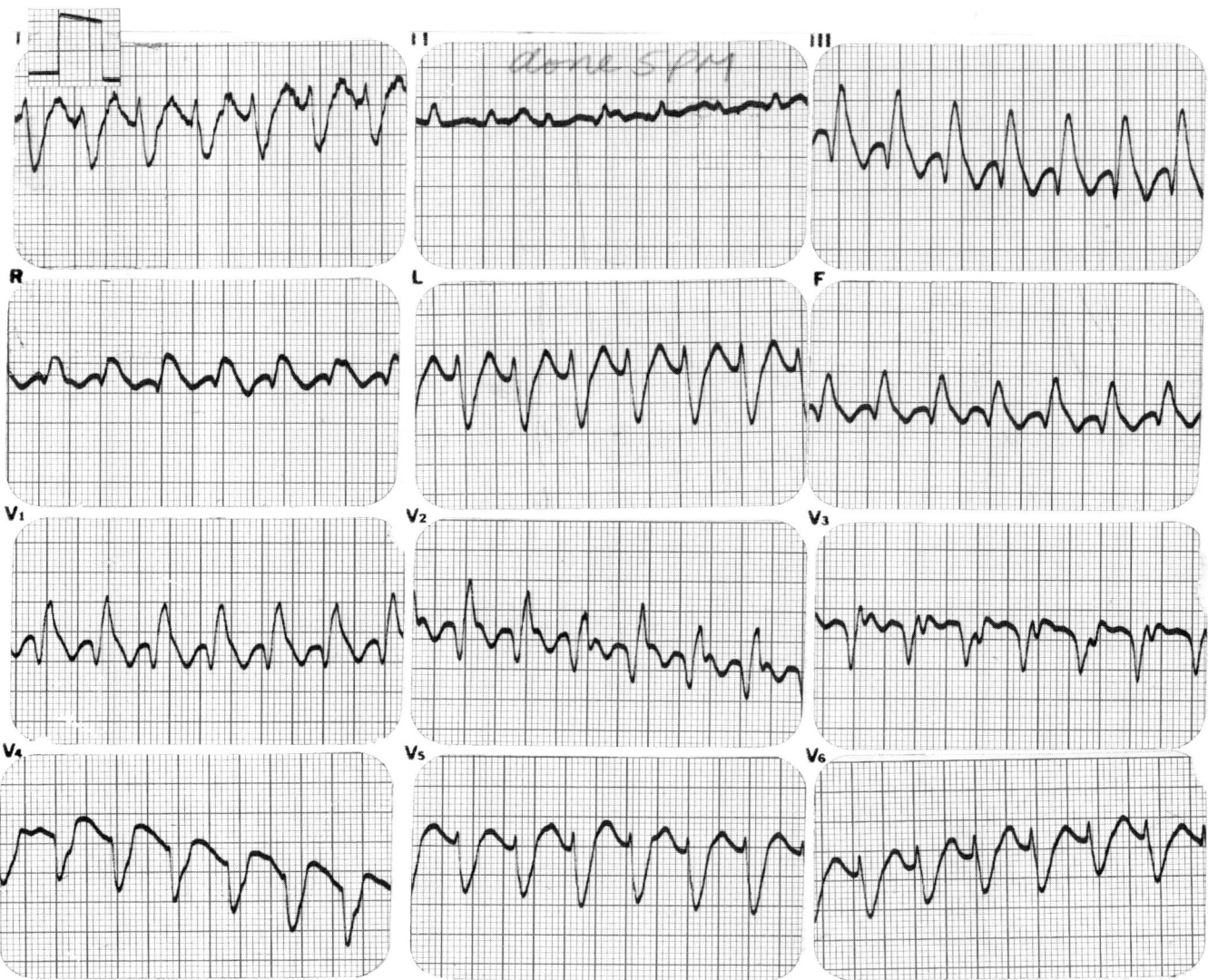

Figure 3-39.

wide than the others of the tachycardia, or fusion beats would favor a ventricular tachycardia, but neither are present in this tracing. We look for capture beats and fusion beats as evidence of atrioventricular dissociation, because in many cases of ventricular tachycardia, AV dissociation is present. Another sign of AV dissociation is finding an independent atrial rhythm. The chances of identifying an independent atrial rhythm even if one is present are small if the QRS and T deflections are large, and in this case they are large in every lead except II. Looking closely at lead II, we can see prominent waves in the baseline that don't seem to be T waves, because they fall at different places in the QRS cycle (heavy arrows, Figure 3-40). Now the question is, are these extra waves P waves going at 100 per minute while the ventricles are beating much faster? We can answer this by making two marks on the edge of a paper corresponding to the arrows. If the paper is moved to the right so that the mark made opposite arrow 1

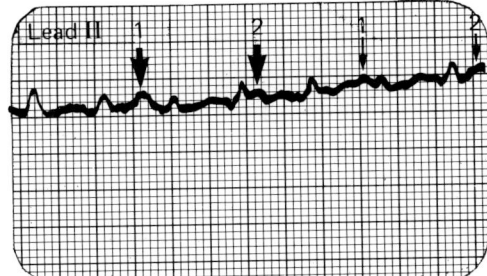

Figure 3-40.

now is at arrow 2, then the other mark points to another unexpected wave (light arrow 1). If we repeat the process, we find yet another unexpected wave (light arrow 2). If we went the other way from the heavy arrows we would come out on top of the first QRS complex, which on close inspection, is taller than all the others in the same lead. Why? Because it is really a QRS plus a P wave. So, we have demonstrated that AV dissociation is indeed present in this case, and that plus the QR pattern is V_1 makes it very likely that this case is a ventricular tachycardia and should be treated as such.

Atrial fibrillation with abnormal intraventricular condition (Figure 5-19) may resemble ventricular tachycardia if the rate is rapid. However, the gross irregularity of the rhythm should immediately eliminate ventricular tachycardia as a diagnostic possibility.

Ventricular fibrillation is perhaps the most dramatic of all cardiac arrhythmias, since it results in immediate cessation of effective pumping. The patient loses consciousness 10 to 12 seconds after ventricular fibrillation starts, and if circulation is not restored within 4 minutes, irreversible brain damage occurs. The electrocardiogram shows a totally chaotic pattern, resembling the atrial pattern of atrial fibrillation except that the waves are larger and no distinct QRS complexes can be identified (Figure 3-41).

No other cardiac rhythm looks like ventricular fibrillation, so diagnosis is usually not a problem. However, a loose electrode may cause artefacts resembling ventricular fibrillation (Figure 1-23, Chapter 1). In such cases, however, the patient will be conscious, and close inspection of the electrocardiogram will show normal QRS complexes among the artefacts.

Ventricular tachycardia and ventricular fibrillation are frequently initiated by premature beats beginning near the crest of the T wave of the previous beat. This period of the cardiac cycle is actually the relatively refractory period of the ventricles, but because it is the part of the cycle in which lethal arrhythmias are most likely to start, it is called the *vulnerable period*. Regardless of its origin (ventricular ectopic focus, supraventricular focus or malfunctioning artificial ventricular pacemaker) a stimulus reaching the ventricles during the vulnerable period is likely to be conducted around more slowly than usual; so the possibility exists for a reentrant ventricular arrhythmia.

The type of arrhythmia that results from stimulation of a ventricle

88 / **Basic Electrocardiography Handbook**

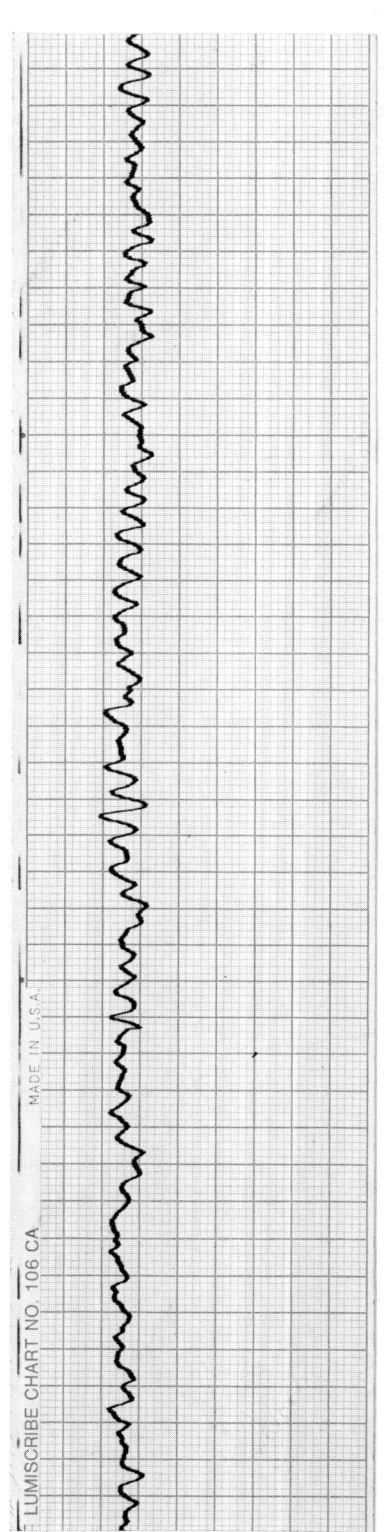

Figure 3-41.

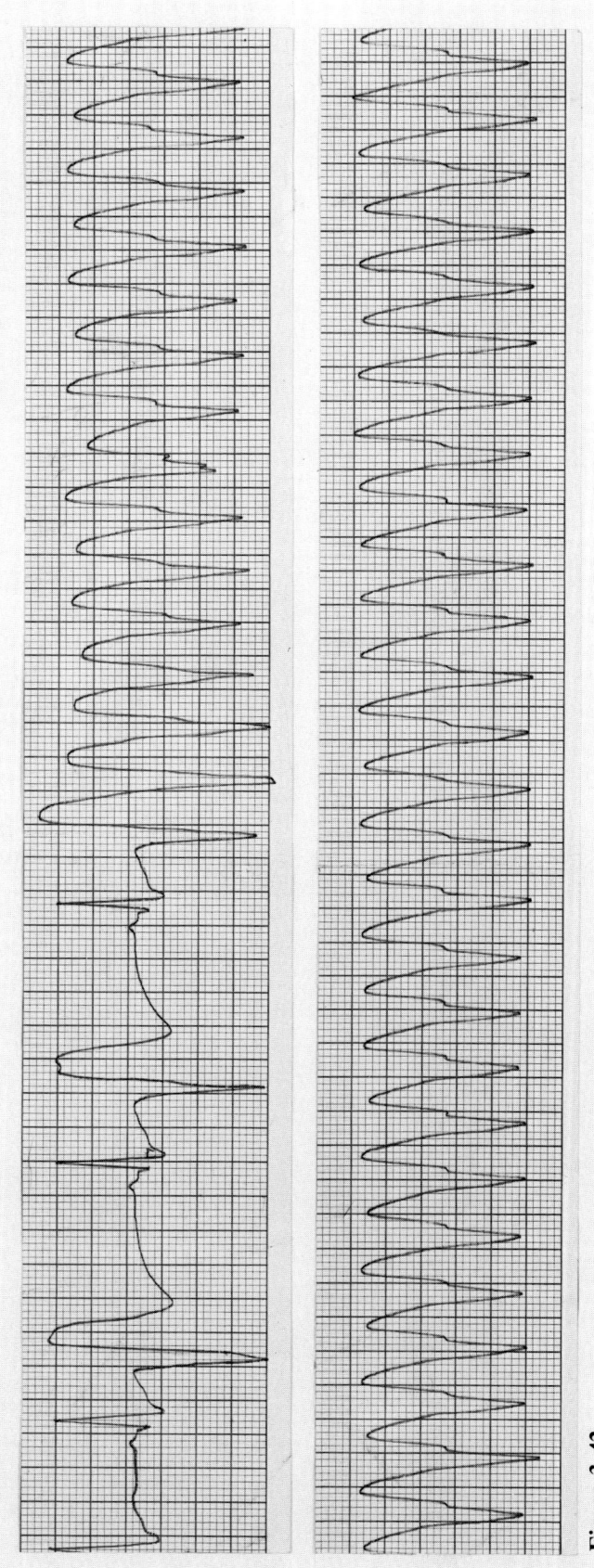

Figure 3-42.

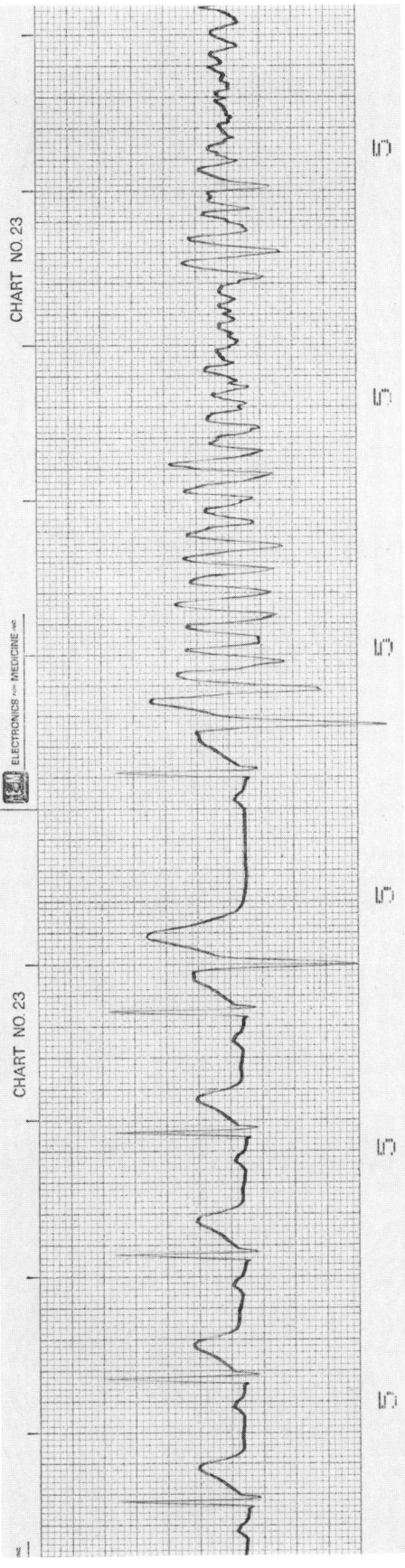

Figure 3-43.

/ Basic Electrocardiography Handbook

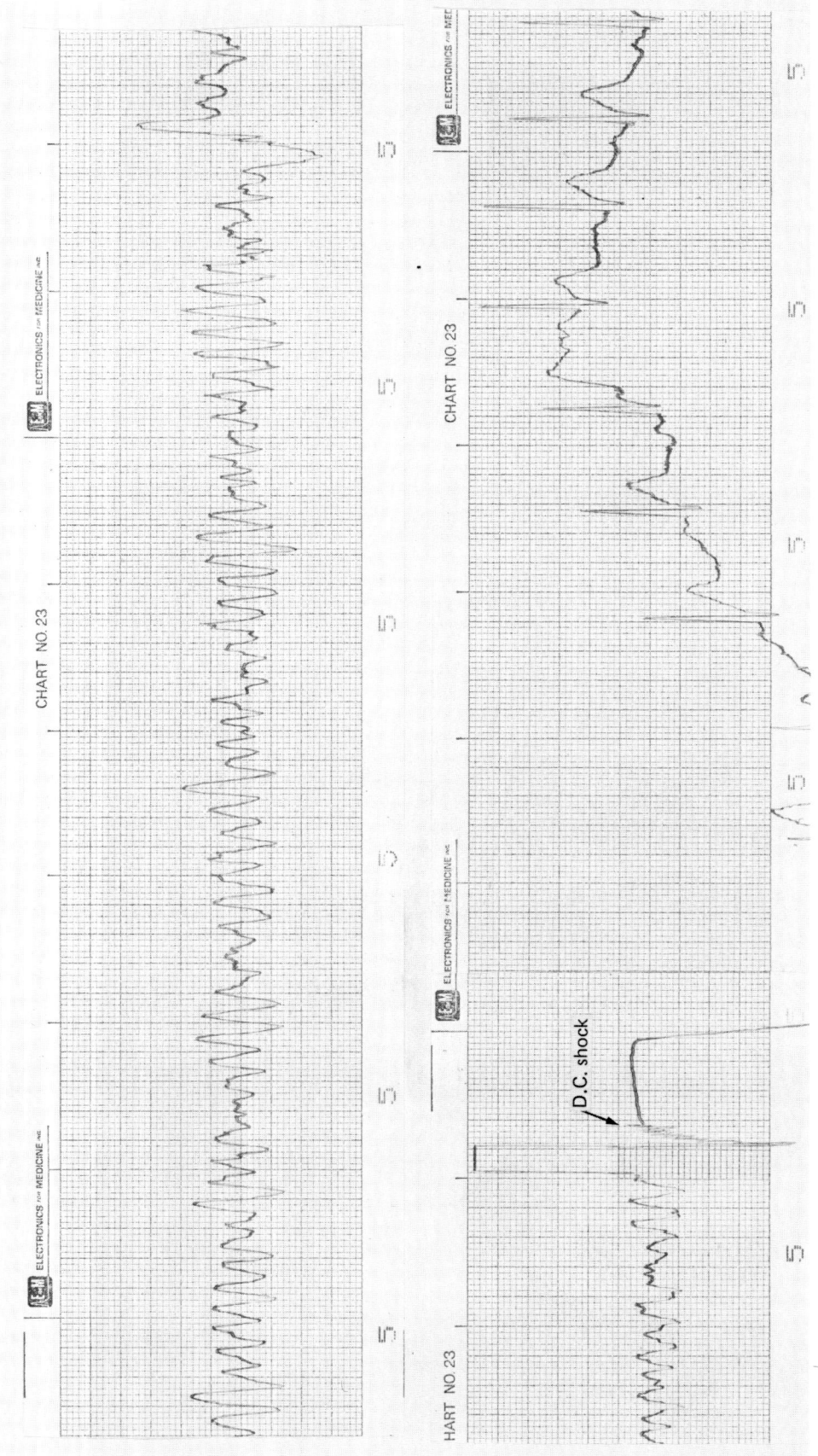

Figure 3-44.

during the vulnerable period depends on the stability of the reentrant circuit. In Figure 3-42, for example, the first two VPB's fell harmlessly on the T wave of the preceding beat. However, the third VPB, coming just a trifle earlier than the other two, initiated a paroxysm of ventricular tachycardia at 184 per minute. The tachycardia persisted until terminated by drug therapy; although the patient's blood pressure fell, there was no loss of consciousness because some cardiac output was maintained. Contrast this with Figure 3-43, where the second VPB in the vulnerable period started unstable ventricular tachycardia which almost immediately degenerated into ventricular fibrillation. Fortunately for this patient, the condition was promptly diagnosed and correctly treated with a direct current shock (Figure 3-44), restoring sinus rhythm, and the patient survived to leave the hospital.

Chapter 4
Myocardial Ischemia and Infarction

ACUTE MYOCARDIAL INFARCTION

Myocardial infarction is what most people mean when they say "heart attack." Acute myocardial infarction is the recent death of heart tissue caused by an inadequate blood supply. The heart is supplied by the coronary arteries; when they become severely narrowed or completely blocked, myocardial infarction may result. An acute myocardial infarction changes the electrical properties of the heart, making it much more susceptible to ventricular tachycardia and fibrillation, a change which accounts for the well-known tendency of people with coronary artery disease to die suddenly. In an intensive care unit or similarly equipped facility these arrhythmias can be treated, but they are usually fatal if they occur anywhere else. Thus in doubtful cases it is best to assume that acute myocardial infarction is present, and (1) immediately begin cardiac monitoring and (2) prepare to treat serious arrhythmias. These measures are the basic ingredients of coronary intensive care; it may be given in an emergency room, a coronary ambulance or a satellite heart station, but in any case should be continued until the patient has been transferred to and stabilized in a coronary intensive care unit, or until the diagnosis of acute myocardial infarction has been definitely excluded.

The electrocardiogram is a very useful tool in diagnosing acute myocardial infarction. Characteristic changes confirm that acute infarction has occurred, and which part of the heart has been affected. However, the absence of typical infarction changes on the electrocardiogram does not rule out acute infarction; for in some cases, particularly in the first few hours when the danger of sudden death is greatest, the changes may be minimal or absent. Therefore, a person with symptoms suggesting acute myocardial infarction should never be sent home from an emergency room or any other medical facility merely because the electrocardiogram is not diagnostic.

Acute myocardial infarction should be suspected in any patient who complains of chest pain lasting more than one-half hour. Usually the pain is in the center of the chest, but it may spread to either side of the chest, to the back, to one or both shoulders or arms and onto the throat and jaws. Patients may describe the pain as burning, squeezing or pressurelike. Sweating, apprehension (including a fear of impending death), shortness of breath, weakness and fainting are additional signs.

Figure 4-1 shows the characteristic electrocardiographic changes of acute *transmural* (literally, across the wall, from endocardium to pericardium but often, just through most of the myocardium) *myocardial infarction*. The earliest change in a current of injury—increased height of the T wave shortly followed by elevation of the ST segment—recorded in leads facing the infarcted area (Figure 4-1, A and B). These changes usually appear minutes to hours after the infarction. While ST segment elevation is recorded in leads facing the infarction, leads facing the opposite side of the heart show ST segment depressions. These are called *reciprocal ST segment depressions* (Figure 4-14, below), and do not indicate myocardial disease in the parts of the heart from which they are recorded. At first the QRS complex is normal; but as muscle cells die, they no longer generate any electrical force, so the R wave becomes smaller,

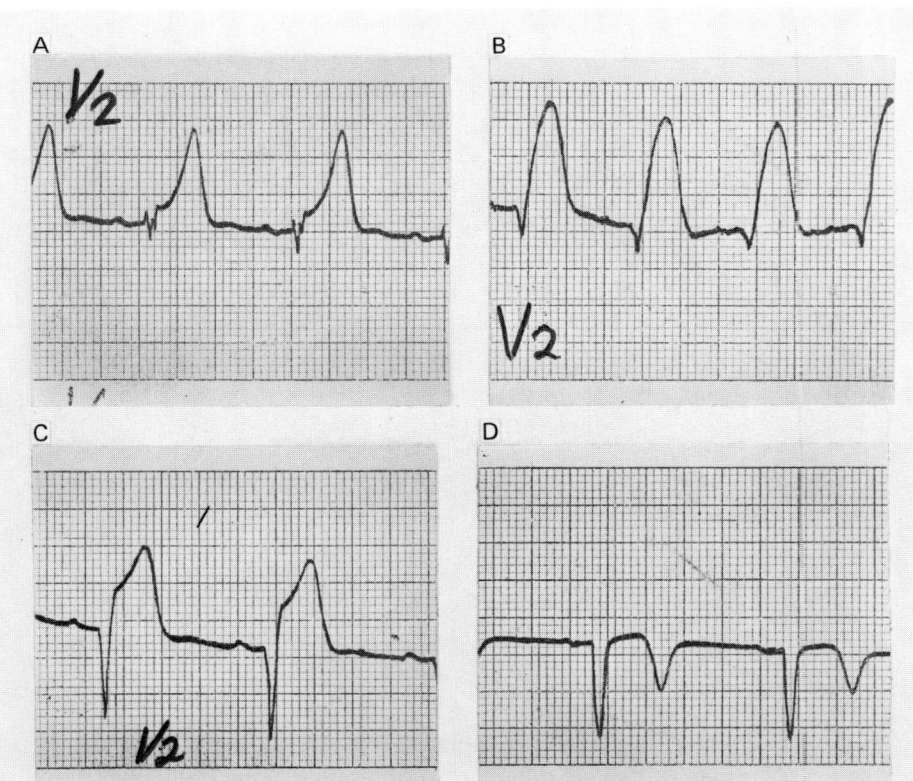

Figure 4-1. Lead V_2—changes after acute transmural infarction. (A) 20 minutes, (B) 1 hour, (C) 3 hours, (D) 11 days.

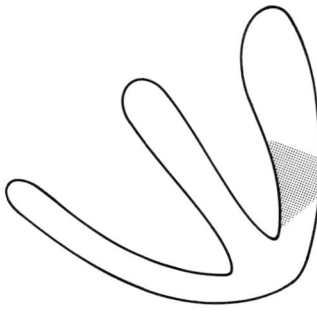 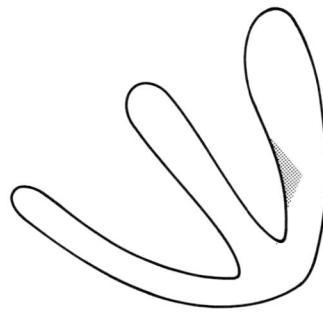

Transmural myocardial infarction — Subendocardial myocardial infarction

Figure 4-2.

or even absent, and a Q wave appears (Figure 4-1, *B*, *C* and *D*). Although small Q waves are found in some leads in normal persons, a Q wave that is longer than .03 second ("*pathological Q wave*") in any lead except AVR almost always means infarction or, if not, some other kind of serious myocardial disease. After the Q wave appears, the T wave becomes inverted, usually symmetrically. This ordinarily occurs within a few days after the infarction. The ST segment returns to normal within two weeks after an uncomplicated infarction, while the T wave gradually becomes deeper (Figure 4-1*D*). It is important to remember that the deepest T inversions may be recorded several weeks after an infarction without any further damage having occurred. Afterwards, the T wave becomes less deeply inverted, and months later may even become upright again. The Q wave may remain or disappear; but even if it disappears, there is still a scar on the heart that has replaced the infarcted muscle tissue.

Small myocardial infarctions may involve less than the entire thickness of the heart wall. These are customarily called *subendocardial myocardial infarctions* (Figure 4-2), although the damage is not always confined to the subendocardial layer. The electrocardiographic changes may be similar to those of transmural infarction except for the absence of pathological Q waves, or they may consist only of T wave inversions.

It is important to remember that many conditions besides subendocardial infarction may cause inverted T waves, so these are nonspecific abnormalities. However, when a patient develops inverted T waves in association with prolonged chest pain and the T waves remain inverted for at least several days, subendocardial infarction has probably occurred.

MYOCARDIAL ISCHEMIA

If blood flow to part of the heart is reduced but not enough to cause acute infarction, it may cause a temporary injury called myocardial ischemia. Myocardial ischemia may occur when coronary blood flow is reduced by a new obstruction, or in patients with previously narrowed coronary arteries when the oxygen needs of the heart increase beyond the limited capacity of the diseased blood vessels. This often happens as the patient overexerts himself or becomes emotionally upset, or when an ectopic tachycardia causes an increase in the heart rate. Recurrent ischemia caused by overexertion or excitement and relieved within minutes by rest, nitroglycerine or similar drugs is called *angina pectoris*. If prolonged or severe, ischemia may lead to infarction, but in most cases cell death does not occur.

Myocardial ischemia causes the same type of chest discomfort as myocardial infarction, but the pain is usually less intense and the duration not as long. Often the pain of ischemia subsides in minutes if the patient rests or takes a nitroglycerine tablet. In other cases, when the pain lasts half an hour or more, it may be difficult to determine whether the patient is suffering from myocardial ischemia or acute infarction. However, since patients are susceptible to the same sudden, potentially fatal arrhythmias during ischemia as during

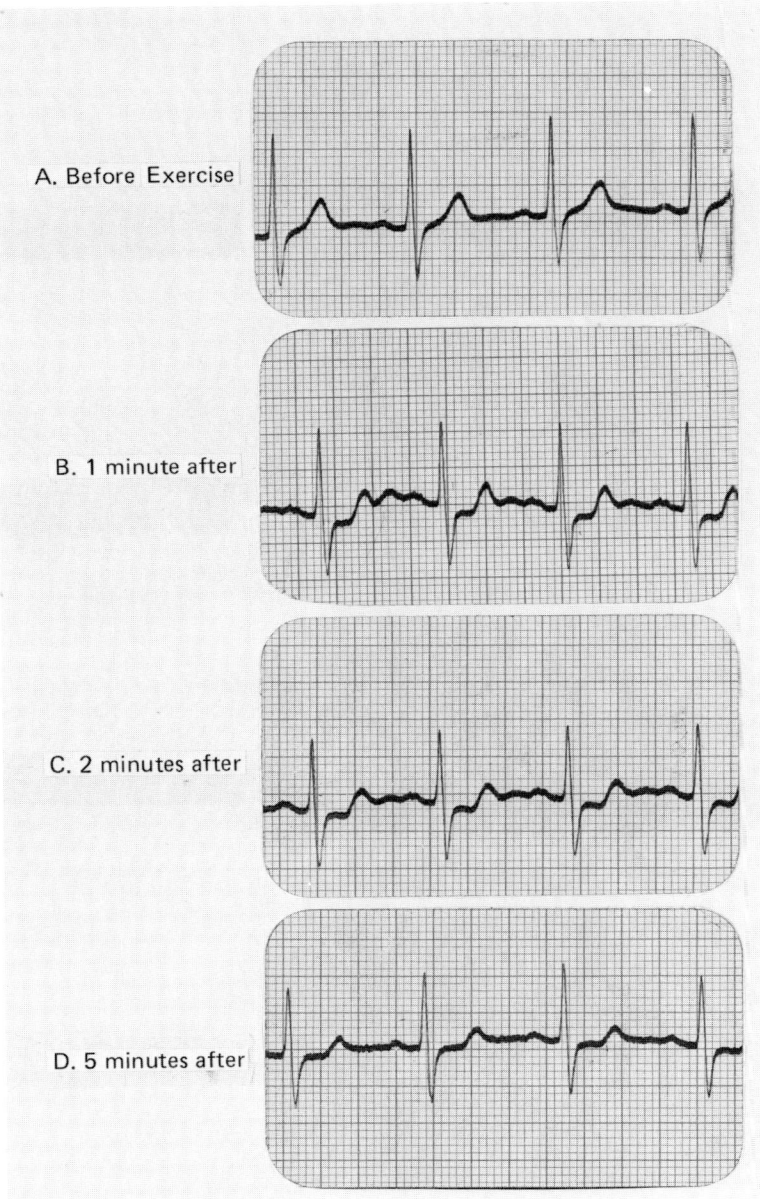

Figure 4-3. Lead V$_5$.

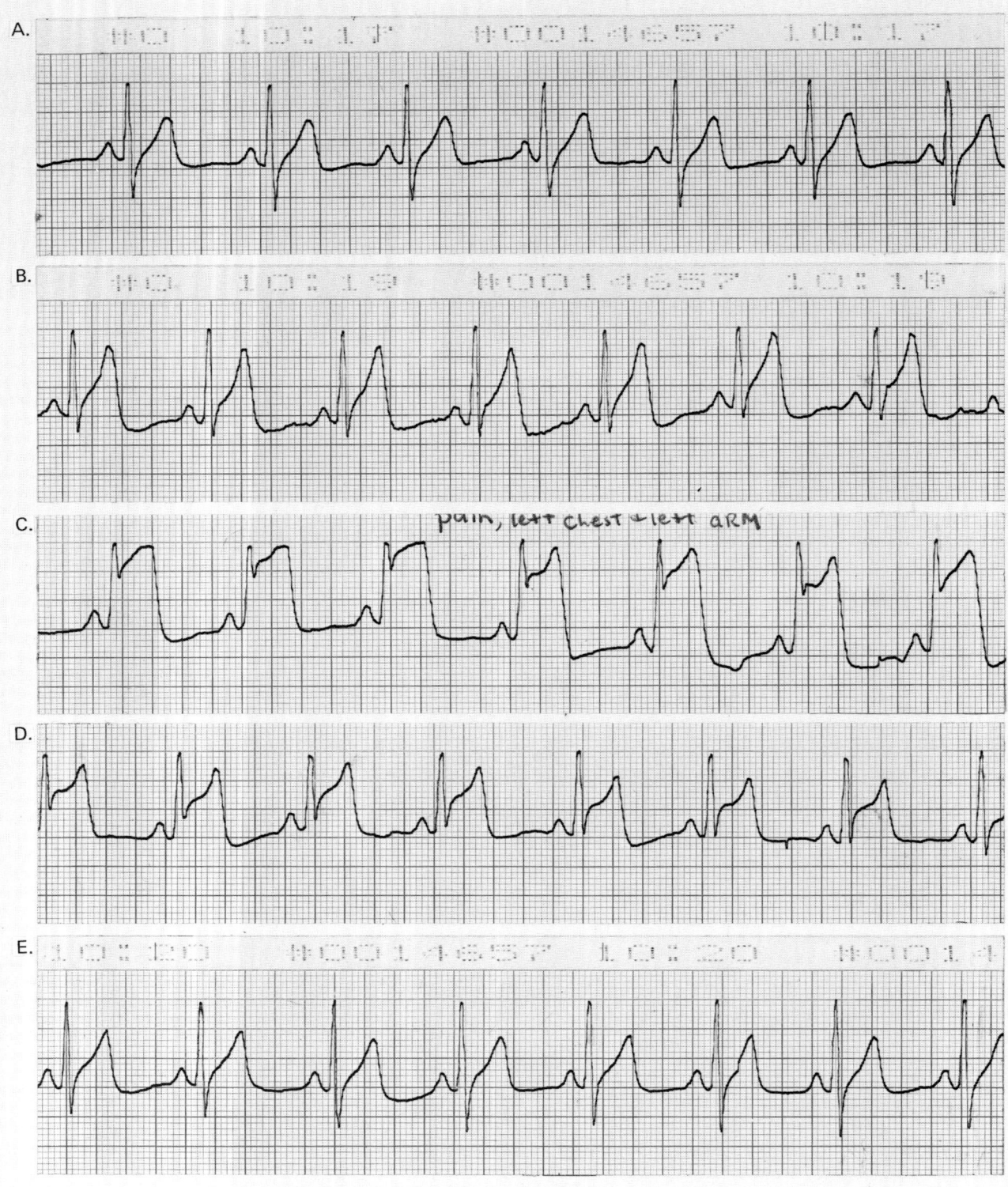

Figure 4-4.

acute infarction, intensive care is also indicated for patients with prolonged myocardial ischemia.

During most instances of myocardial ischemia, the ischemia is limited to the subendocardial layers. This causes ST segment depressions to appear, or become deeper in leads facing the ischemic zone. When the ischemia subsides, the ST segments return to where they were before. Figure 4-3 shows ischemic changes brought on by exercise in a patient with angina pectoris. Before exercise (A) the ST segments were normal. One minute after exercise, and while the patient was experiencing chest tightness (B), the ST segments were depressed by almost 2 mm as compared to the baseline, the T-P segment. Two minutes after exercise (C) there was hardly any change; but by 5 minutes after exercise (D), the ischemic changes were greatly diminished, and later they disappeared altogether.

An uncommon, but spectacular, type of myocardial ischemia is known as *Prinzmetal's angina*. Most, if not all cases, are caused by spasm of one or more major coronary arteries. Therefore, instead of producing the usual subendocardial ischemia, this sudden, severe coronary artery narrowing produces transmural ischemia with electrocardiographic changes just like acute transmural infarction, except that they go away when the ischemia subsides. Figure 4-4 shows monitor strips recorded from a patient with Prinzmetal's angina. Strip A, recorded at 10:17, shows normal ST segments and T waves. At 10:19 (strip B) there is slight elevation of the J point and increased height of the T waves. Notice the similarity to Figure 4-1A. Later (strip C), when the patient felt pain in the chest and left arm, there is marked ST segment elevation. Still at 10:19 (strip D) the ST segments begin to come down, and by 10:20 (strip E) they have returned to normal. Although this patient remained in sinus rhythm throughout the attack, sometimes Prinzmetal's angina is accompanied by dangerous ventricular arrhythmias or heart block.

LOCALIZATION OF MYOCARDIAL INFARCTION

The overwhelming majority of deaths from acute myocardial infarction are either electrical deaths (caused by an abnormal rhythm or a conduction disturbance) or pump failure deaths (where myocardial damage is so extensive that the heart cannot pump enough blood to sustain normal function in other vital organs of the body). Modern coronary intensive care can prevent most electrical deaths if pump failure is not present, and also in some cases with pump failure. However, the death rate remains very high in cases with severe pump failure. Since certain complications are more common with infarctions affecting particular parts of the heart, knowing the location of the infarction helps one to anticipate problems.

It is customary to identify infarctions by the part of the left ventricle that is involved, for the right ventricle is not often affected by acute infarction, perhaps since it does less work and so requires less oxygen and other nutrients than the left ventricle. *Inferior myocardial infarction* involves the lower part of the left ventricle. Telltale changes are seen in leads which face the inferior wall of the left ventricle—

III, F and frequently II as well. Uncomplicated inferior infarctions are usually not large, so pump failure is infrequent; if electrical deaths can be prevented, these patients usually do very well. Figure 4-5 shows a typical electrocardiogram from a patient with a recent inferior infarction. There are QR patterns in II, III and F. Although in II the Q is only .02 second in duration, leads III and F both have pathological Q waves. All three leads also show symmetrically inverted T waves.

Anterior wall infarctions may involve part or all of the front part of the left ventricle, so electrocardiographic signs of infarction appear in one or more of the V leads. As a rule, anterior wall infarctions are larger than those affecting the inferior wall, so pump failure is a more frequent complication and the overall mortality rate is higher. Another important difference is that conduction disturbances in anterior wall infarctions usually result from damage to the bundle

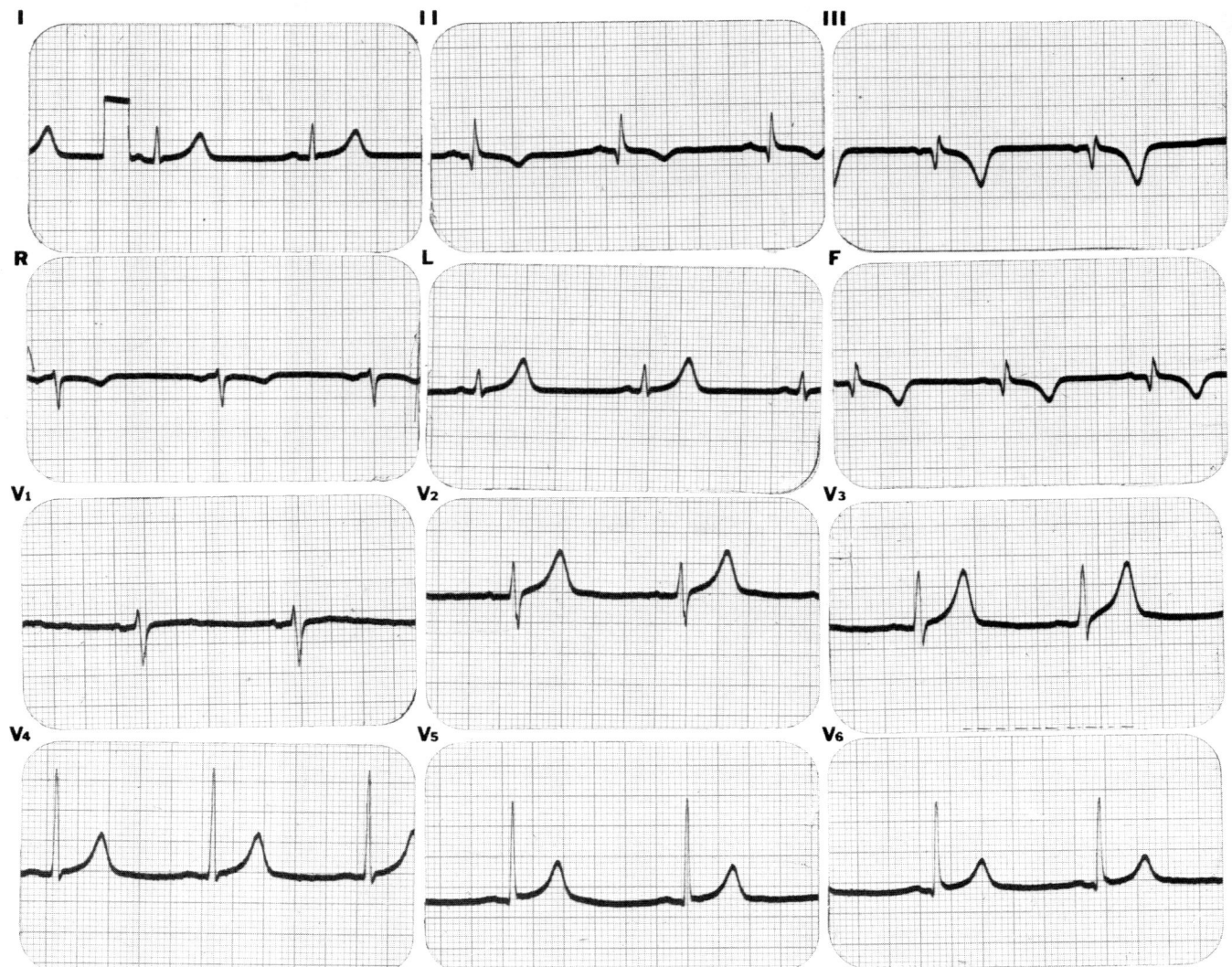

Figure 4-5.

branches, while in inferior or posterior infarctions the AV node may be damaged but the bundle branches are almost always spared.

Anterior wall infarctions are often further classified as anteroseptal, anterior (apical or midanterior), anterolateral and extensive anterior, according to which leads show damage. The localizing criteria for myocardial infarction are summarized in Table 4-1. With respect to the precise diagnosis of anterior wall infarctions, the following points should be emphasized: (1) If V_1 shows evidence of infarction, then the diagnosis is anteroseptal infarction unless the damage extends to V_5 or beyond, in which case the correct diagnosis is extensive anterior infarction. (2) In addition to the Q waves in V_1 seen in anteroseptal infarction, damage to the interventricular septum often causes loss of normal left-to-right septal depolarization so that a septal Q wave is not recorded in V_6. (3) If V_5 and V_6 show evidence of infarction, the diagnosis is anterolateral infarction unless the damage extends as far to the right as V_2, in which case it is an extensive anterior infarction.

Small infarctions may damage only the upper lateral wall of the left ventricle (*high lateral myocardial infarction*). In such cases, only lead L may show the signs of infarction, or they may appear in leads I and L. Most of the time, though, lateral wall damage is not

Table 4-1. Electrocardiographic Localization of Myocardial Infarction

Location	Leads showing evidence of infarction
Inferior	F
	III, F
	II, III, F
Inferolateral	same + V_6 (I, L)
Anteroseptal	V_1
	V_1, V_2
	V_1, V_2, V_3
	V_1, V_2, V_3, V_4
Anterior (apical)	V_3 or V_4
	V_3, V_4
	V_2, V_3, V_4
Anterolateral	V_5, V_6 (I, L)
	V_4, V_5, V_6 (I, L)
	V_3, V_4, V_5, V_6 (I, L)
Extensive anterior	V_2–V_6 (I, L)
	V_1–V_6 (I, L)
	V_1–V_5 (I, L)
High lateral	L
	I, L
Posterior	V_2 (R taller than S and at least .04 sec)
	V_2, V_1 (R taller than S and at least .04 sec)
	T wave usually upright, V_1
Posterolateral	same + V_6 (I, L)

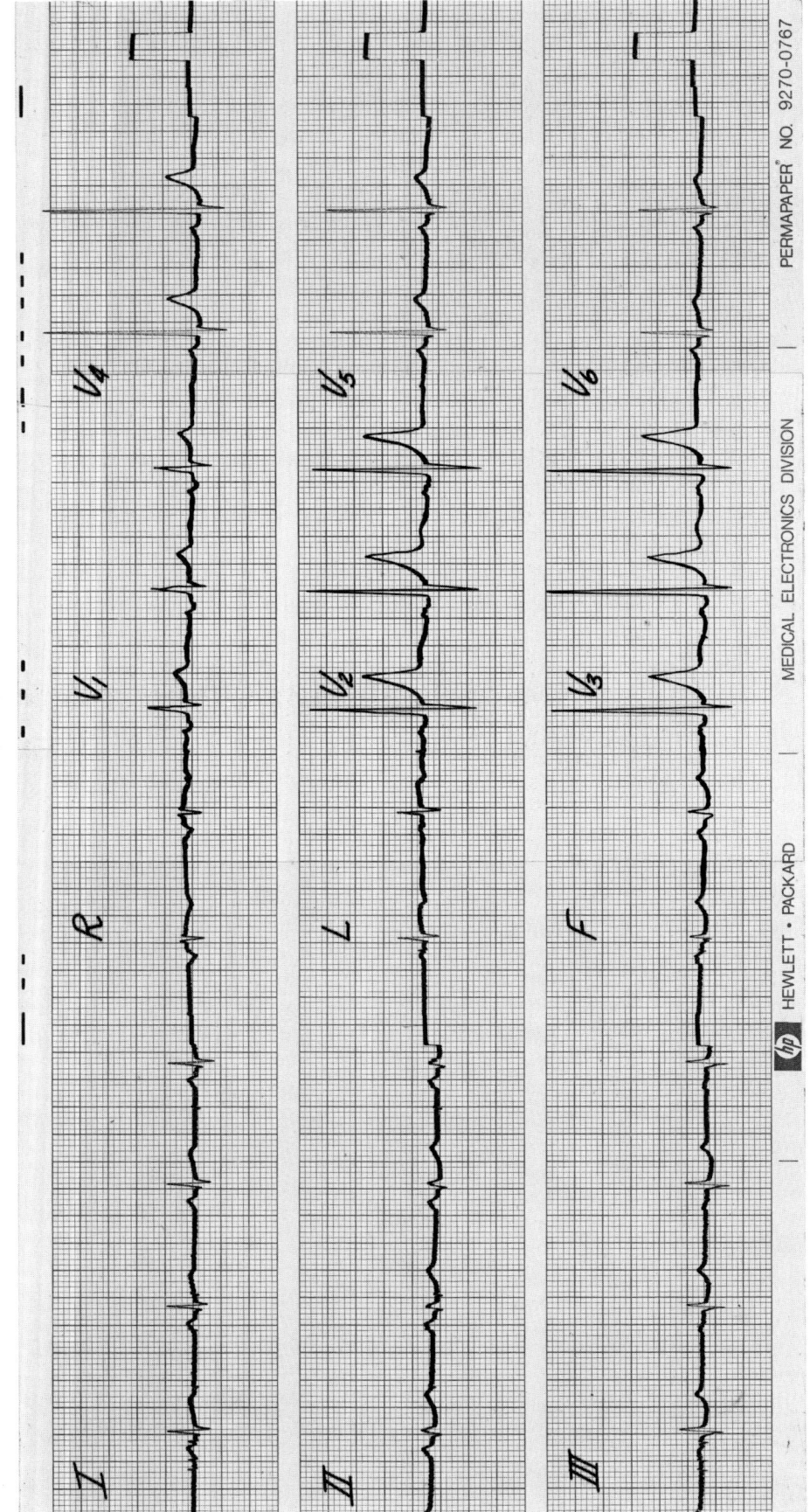

Figure 4-6.

isolated but extends to the anterior wall (anterolateral infarction), the inferior wall (inferolateral infarction) or the posterior wall (posterolateral infarction), or even to several of these areas (inferoposterolateral, for example). These combined infarctions are diagnosed when changes in I, L or V_6 are combined with changes of inferior or posterior infarction.

Probably the most difficult transmural infarction to diagnose is one involving the back wall of the left ventricle (*posterior myocardial infarction*), because there are no electrocardiographic leads that overlie this part of the heart. However, the loss of electrical forces going posteriorly causes the anterior forces to appear larger, particularly in leads V_1 and V_2. Since these leads face the opposite side of the heart from the infarcted area, they show changes opposite to those expected in leads facing an infarction. In other words, instead of a Q wave appearing, the R wave becomes wider and taller. From the diagnostic standpoint, it is fortunate that isolated posterior infarction is uncommon. It usually accompanies either inferior or lateral wall infarction. Indeed, the electrocardiographic diagnosis of isolated posterior infarction is not a safe diagnosis unless there is other evidence of infarction, such as prolonged chest pain, elevated myocardial enzymes, definite sequential electrocardiographic changes from day to day and so on.

Figure 4-6 is an electrocardiogram from a patient with an old inferior and a recent posterior infarction. The small Q in II and the pathological Q waves in III and F indicate inferior infarction. The T waves are upright in those leads, probably because the infarction is many months old. The R waves are .04 second wide and taller than the S waves in V_1 and V_2.

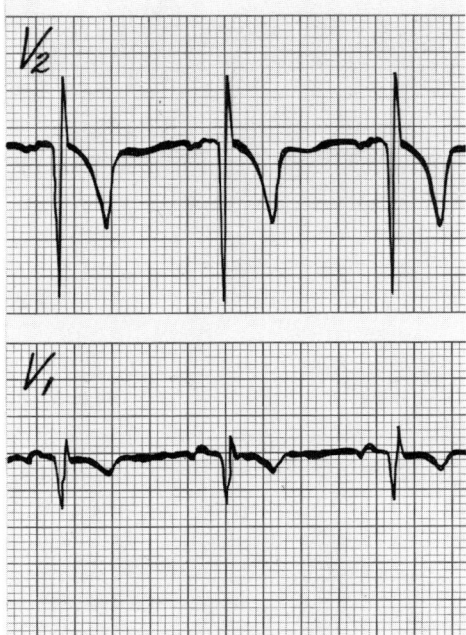

Figure 4-7. Leads V_1 and V_2 from Figure 4-6 drawn upside down.

The T waves are upright in both leads. Remember, V_1 and V_2 are on the opposite side of the heart from the posterior infarction, so the electrocardiographic findings are exactly the opposite of those expected in leads facing the infarction. To illustrate this point, Figure 4-7 shows leads V_1 and V_2 of Figure 4-6 drawn upside down. Shown this way, the changes are typical of recent infarction.

Simplified Localization of Myocardial Infarction

If you find the classification of myocardial infarction as outlined in Table 4-1 too complicated or too hard to remember, you can settle for distinguishing between inferior and anterior wall infarctions. Although such a simple classification lacks the precision of the more detailed classification, it is good enough to help you anticipate complications. If there is evidence of infarction in I, L or any of the V leads, call it anterior wall infarction. If there is evidence of either inferior or posterior infarction or both, as listed in Table 4-1, call it an inferior wall infarction.

Review of Myocardial Infarction Localization

Cases 1–6 (Figures 4-8–4-13) are electrocardiograms recorded from patients with recent or old myocardial infarctions. Analyze each one, and localize the infarction. Refer to Table 4-1 if necessary. Be sure to note any associated conduction disorders.

Case 1 (Figure 4-8). There are pathological Q waves in leads I, L and V_{1-5}. ST elevations are present in leads I, L and V_{1-4}, and T inversions in leads I, L and V_{1-6}. There should be no difficulty in diagnosing this as an extensive anterior infarction.

Case 2 (Figure 4-9). Before rushing to the QRS complexes be sure to check the PR interval. It is .24 second, so there is first degree AV block. Now you can look at the QRS complexes. They are normal. Specifically, there are no pathological Q waves. The ST segments are also not remarkable. However, the T waves in L are deeply and symmetrically inverted, and those in I are shallowly inverted. If we knew that this patient formerly had a normal electrocardiogram and in the interval had prolonged chest pain, we could diagnose high lateral, subendocardial infarction. Without that sort of information, we would have to interpret this as "nonspecific T abnormalities, consistent with high lateral subendocardial infarction." In this particular case, serial electrocardiographic changes after prolonged chest pain confirmed that acute infarction had occurred.

Case 3 (Figure 4-10). Pathologic Q waves are present in leads I, II, L, F and V_6. There are ST segment depressions in I, II, V_5 and V_6 and inverted T waves in leads I, L and V_6. What does this add up to? First of all, exclude the ST segment depressions from consideration when you localize the infarction. Since Q waves are present, this is a transmural infarction. ST segment depression is not a sign of transmural infarction at any stage; it may be seen with subendocardial infarction,

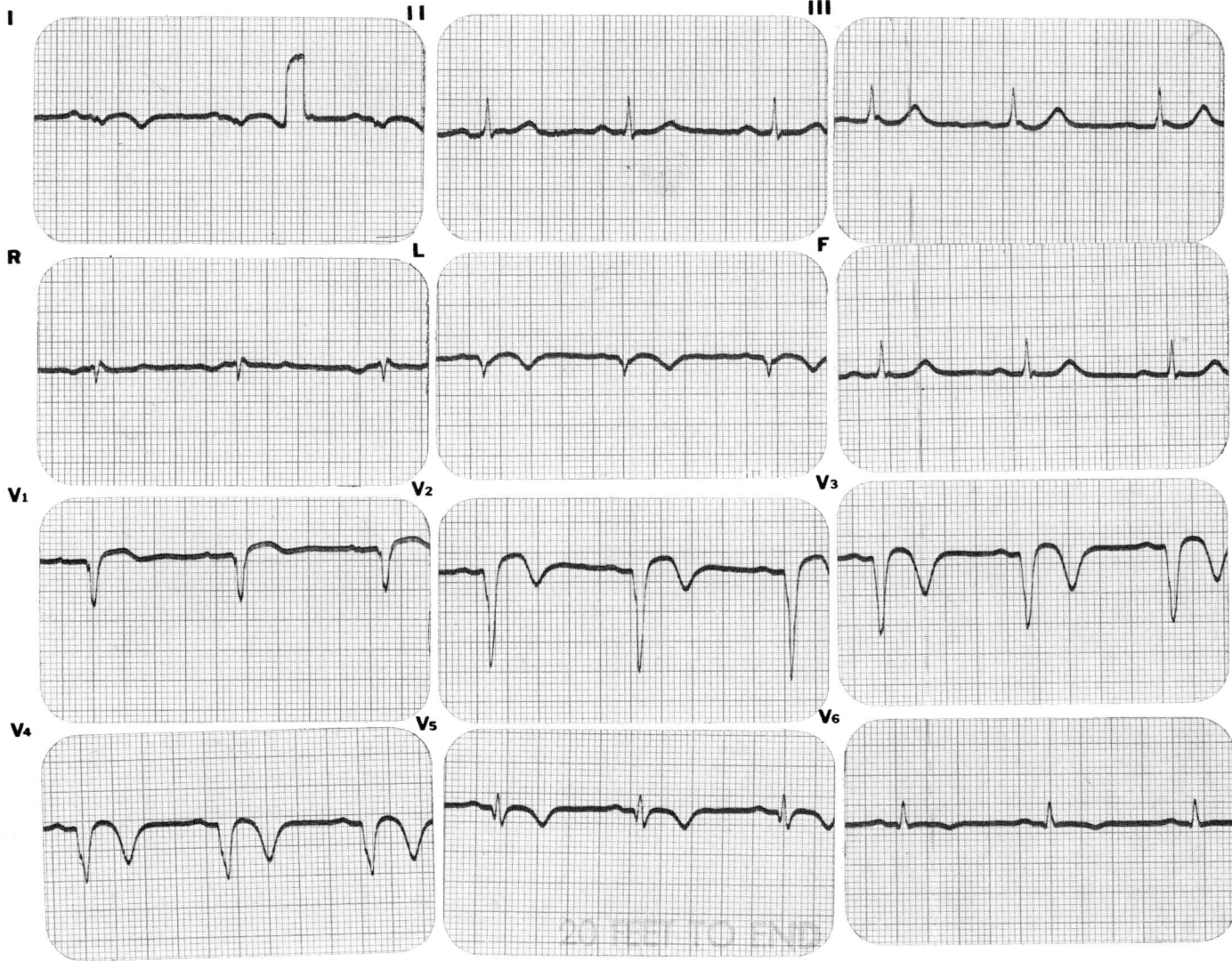

Figure 4-8. Case 1.

but it is a nonspecific finding. On the other hand, inverted T waves are seen with transmural infarctions after the first few days (see above, Figure 4-1). So, there is evidence of infarction in I, II, L, F and V_6. Leads II and F indicate inferior wall infarction, while I, L and V_6 show lateral wall involvement. I hope you also noticed that in V_1 and V_2 the R wave is taller than the S wave. Furthermore, the R in V_2 is more than .04 second in duration, and the T in V_1 is upright. All of these findings indicate posterior wall involvement. Therefore, the answer is inferoposterolateral infarction.

Case 4 (Figure 4-11). There is normal sinus rhythm, but with a PR interval of .24 second; therefore, first degree AV block is present. The QRS complexes are wide (.16 second) with a QR pattern in V_1 and wide S waves in V_6, indicating right bundle branch block. Now looking for pathological Q waves, we see them in leads V_1, V_2 and V_3.

104 / Basic Electrocardiography Handbook

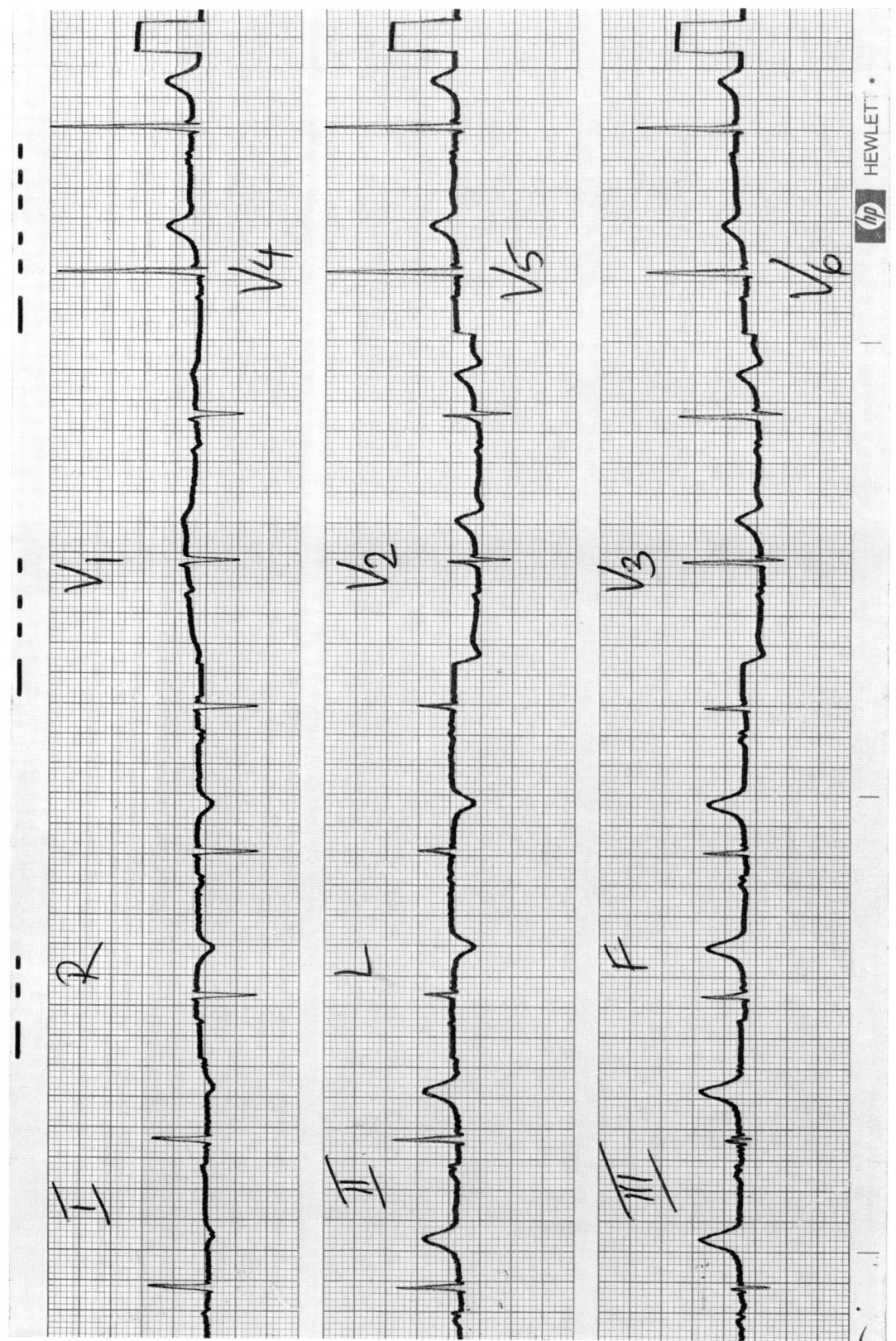

Figure 4-9. Case 2.

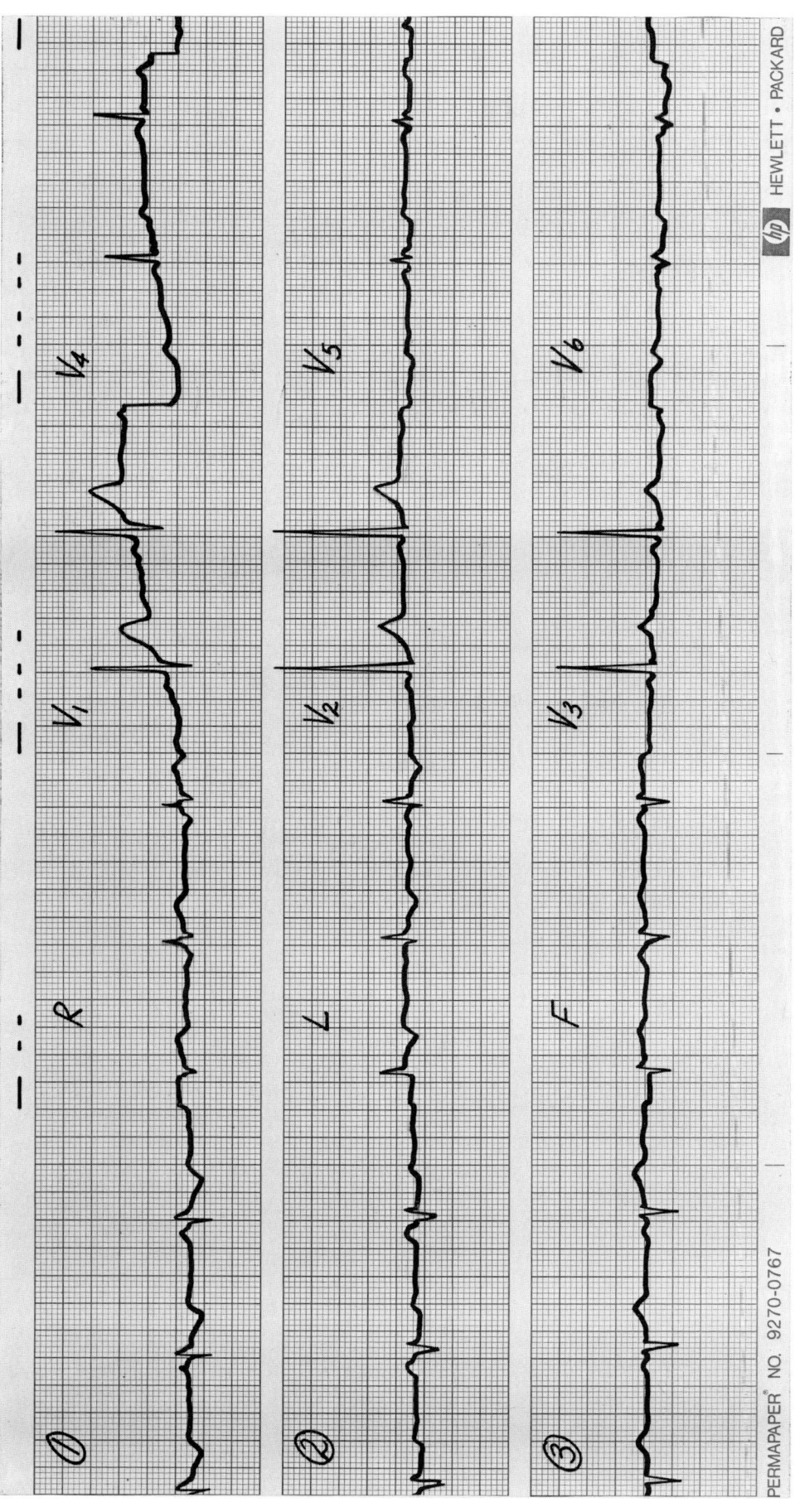

Figure 4-10. Case 3.

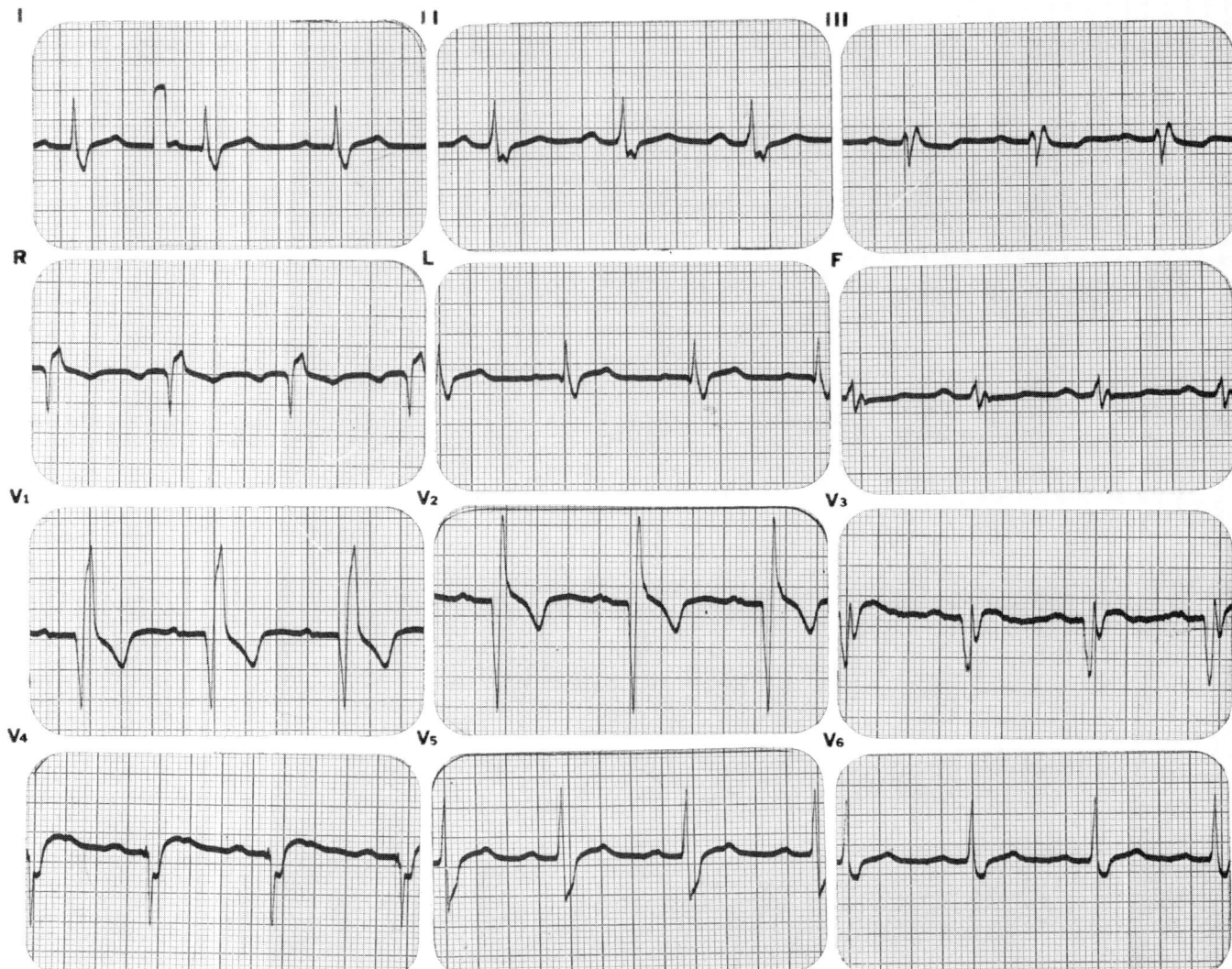

Figure 4-11. Case 4.

In addition, the R wave in lead V_4, which ought to be quite tall, is almost nonexistent in this case. However, the R wave in V_5 looks all right. In V_6 there is no septal Q wave. Since there is evidence of infarction in leads V_{1-4}, this is an anteroseptal infarction. Notice that even though right bundle branch block is present, coexistent infarction can be easily diagnosed.

Case 5 (Figure 4-12). There is a small Q in lead I. By itself, it would not be diagnostic of infarction, but we must consider the company it keeps—in this case, slight ST segment elevation followed by an inverted T wave. Lead L has a pathological Q wave followed by the same ST and T abnormalities. Small Q waves are present in leads V_{3-6}, again followed by elevated ST segments and inverted T waves. With evidence of infarction in leads I, L and V_{3-6}, this is an anterolateral infarction.

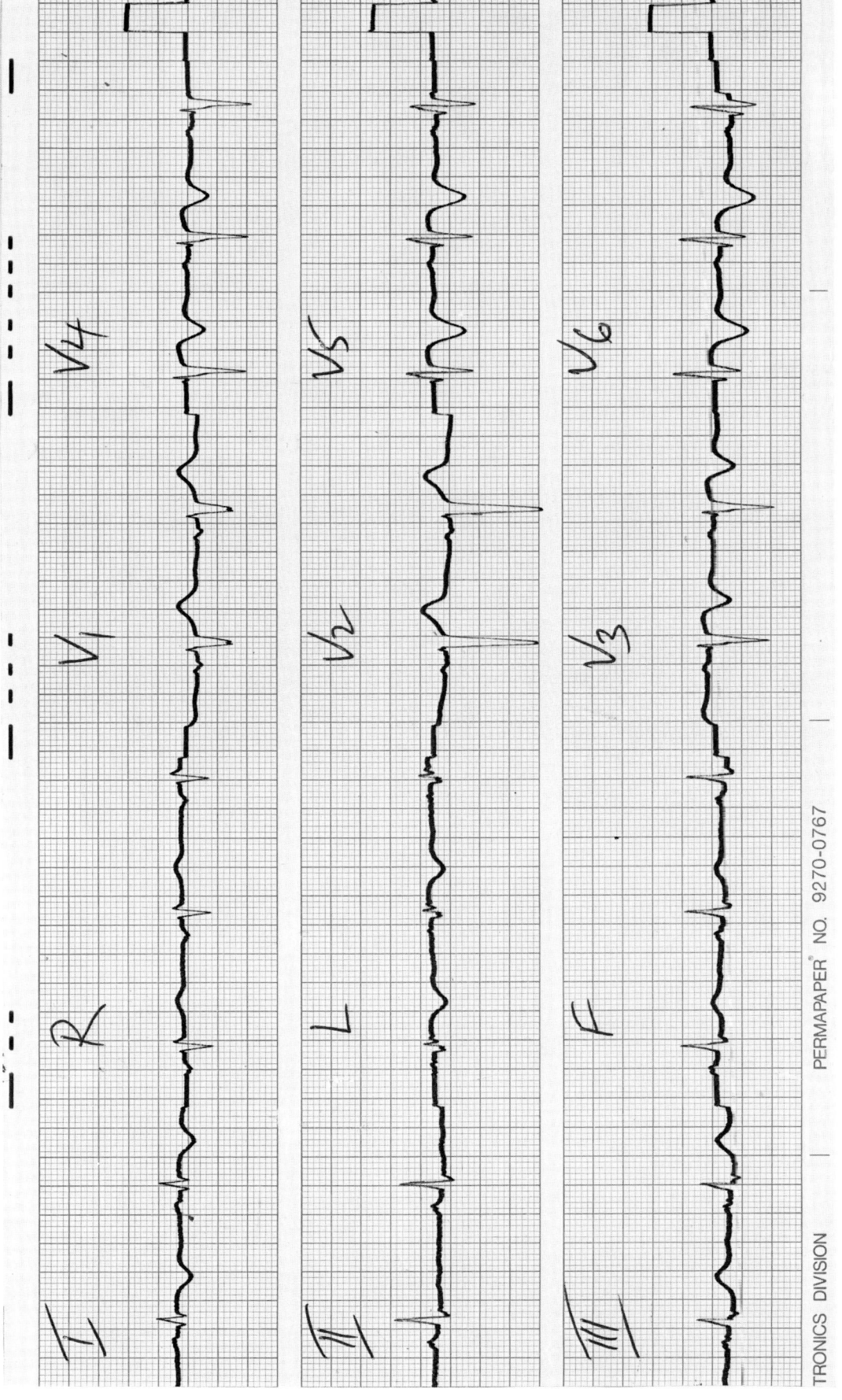

Figure 4-12. Case 5.

108 / Basic Electrocardiography Handbook

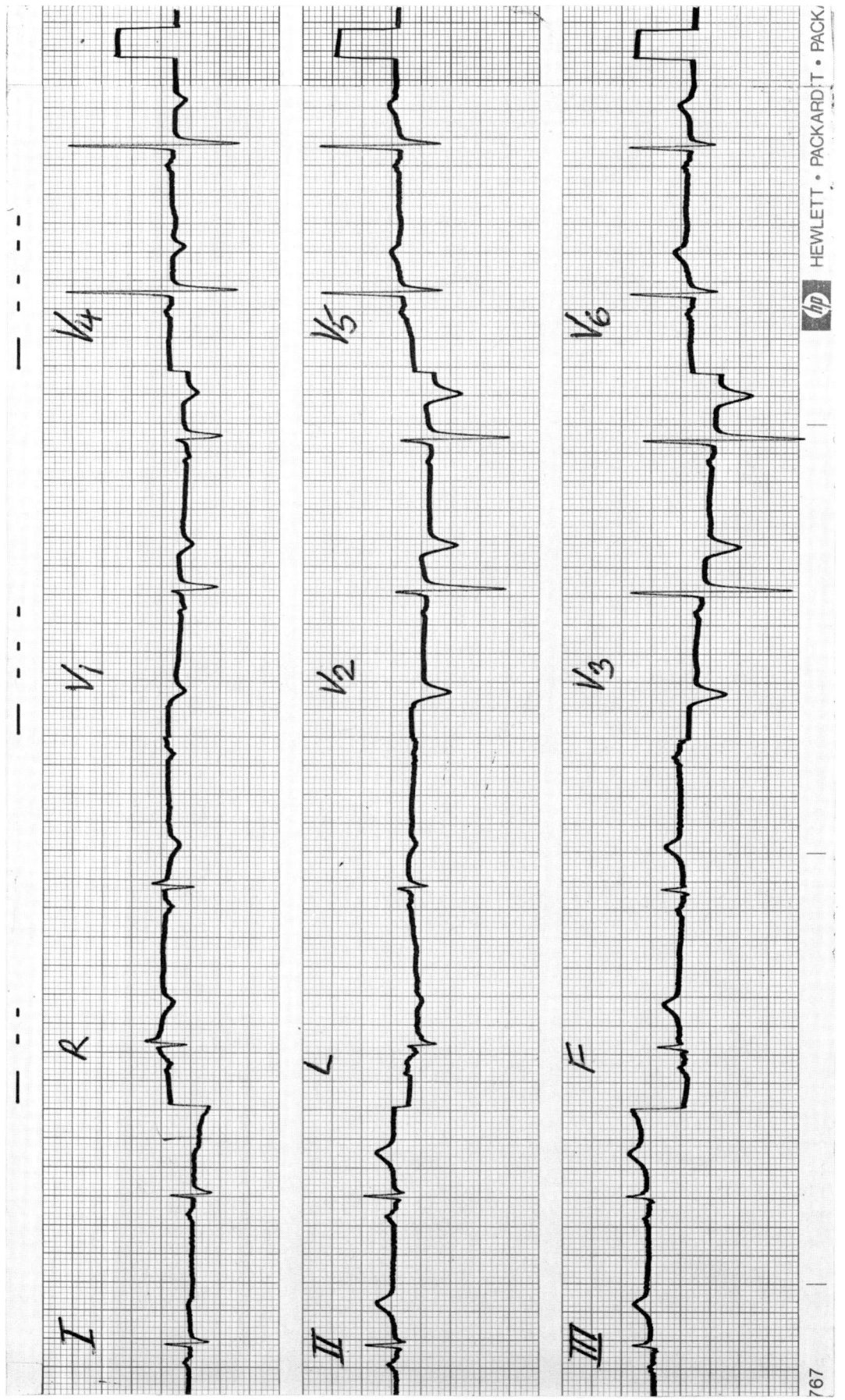

Figure 4-13. Case 6.

Case 6 (Figure 4-13). The QRS complexes do not look abnormal. There is a small Q wave in lead III, but the ST segment and T wave are normal in that lead, and there is no evidence of infarction in F; so inferior infarction cannot be diagnosed from this tracing. Major ST segment and T wave abnormalities are present, however. There are ST segment elevations in leads V_1 and V_2, deep, symmetrical T inversions in leads V_2 and V_3 and smaller T inversions in V_1 and V_4. Therefore, this is another case of anteroseptal infarction; but, without Q waves, it is a subendocardial, anteroseptal infarction.

CONDUCTION DISORDERS IN MYOCARDIAL INFARCTION

Since an acute myocardial infarction may include damage to the AV node or the bundle branches, any of the conduction disorders described in Chapter 2 may appear. Recognition of these disorders is important, since frequently a decision must be made as to whether to use drugs or insert a pacemaker to stabilize the heart rhythm. This decision frequently hinges on the type of block identified and the location of the infarction.

Inferior and posterior infarction usually result from obstruction of the posterior descending coronary artery. Since the artery to the AV node is a branch of this artery, conduction disturbances caused by malfunction of the AV node are characteristic of inferior wall infarction. Bundle branch block is quite uncommon. The following conduction disorders are seen in inferior infarction, frequently in sequence over a period of hours to days: first degree AV block, type I second degree AV block and complete AV block with junctional escape rhythm. Most of the time, the escaping junctional pacemaker is accelerated, so that instead of a simple type I second degree AV block the block is combined with accelerated junctional escape beats, and instead of complete AV block there is AV dissociation.

The important point about conduction disorders in inferior infarction is that the junctional pacemaker is usually fast enough to maintain an adequate cardiac output and stable enough that there is almost no chance of sudden asystole, so that unless the heart rate falls below 50, or there is evidence of pump failure (low blood pressure, congestive heart failure or shock) or ventricular ectopic rhythms, a pacemaker is not required. Furthermore, since damage to the AV node in inferior infarction is almost always temporary, the conduction disorders usually last for only a few days, more or less. For these reasons, conduction disorders are not usually a very serious complication of inferior infarction, and the likelihood of a patient's dying from acute inferior infarction complicated by second or third degree AV block or AV dissociation is only slightly greater than that for a patient with an inferior infarction without conduction problems.

It is a very different situation when conduction disorders appear in acute anterior wall infarction. Here, the AV node is usually spared, but one or more of the fascicles are damaged by the infarction. In many cases the damage is permanent. If more than one fascicle is damaged, it indicates a large area of infarction; indeed, about 50% of patients with anterior infarction and bifascicular block die because of pump failure. In cases of complete heart block with anterior infarction the expected mortality is close to 90% even if the rhythm is controlled by a pacemaker. The fact that most of these patients are destined to die from pump failure limits the potential for saving lives by timely pacemaker insertion. As a result, there is some controversy at present regarding the indications for pacing patients with anterior infarction and conduction disorders. Since the risk of pacemaker insertion is minimal if the operator is experienced, I personally favor the use of pacemakers in many of these patients; for no harm is being done to those who will die anyway from pump failure, and an occasional person is being saved from death resulting from complete heart block.

Unlike patients with inferior infarction and heart block, patients with anterior wall infarction do not progress from first to second to third degree block. Frequently, they go abruptly from normal atrioventricular conduction (no PR prolongation) to complete heart block. Since idioventricular pacemakers are often unstable, the complete heart block may be accompanied by asystole. Therefore it is desirable to have a pacemaker in place before complete heart block develops.

Complete heart block in anterior infarction is trifascicular block. It is usually preceded by bifascicular block, although the interval between the appearance of bifascicular block and complete heart block may be as short as a few hours. For this reason, recognition of a new bifascicular block in an acute anterior infarction identifies a patient at high risk of developing complete heart block, and one in whom the use of a pacemaker should be strongly considered.

Figures 4-14 and 4-15 A and B are electrocardiograms taken from two patients with acute myocardial infarction complicated by conduction disorders. Analyze them, then answer these questions: (1) Where is the infarction? (2) What is the conduction disorder? (3) Is the risk of death in pump failure great or small? (4) Should this patient be treated with a pacemaker?

Figure 4-14 shows a regular sinus rhythm of 92 per minute with an irregular ventricular rhythm. However, the QRS complexes are narrow in all leads, so they must be of supraventricular origin. The rhythm is best analyzed in the lead II rhythm strip at the bottom, which shows (reading from left to right) that the first P wave is followed by a QRS complex with a PR interval of .20 second and the second by a QRS with a PR of .28 second, while the third P is not conducted at all. The fourth P wave is conducted with PR interval of .18 second, and so the sequence continues. Since some P waves are conducted while others are blocked, this is second degree AV block. Since the PR intervals change, and the RR intervals around the blocked P are less than twice the shortest RR, this is type I second degree AV block.

Turning now to an analysis of the QRS complexes, we can see small Q waves in leads III and F. By themselves, these small Q waves are only suspicious, but in combination with the marked ST segment

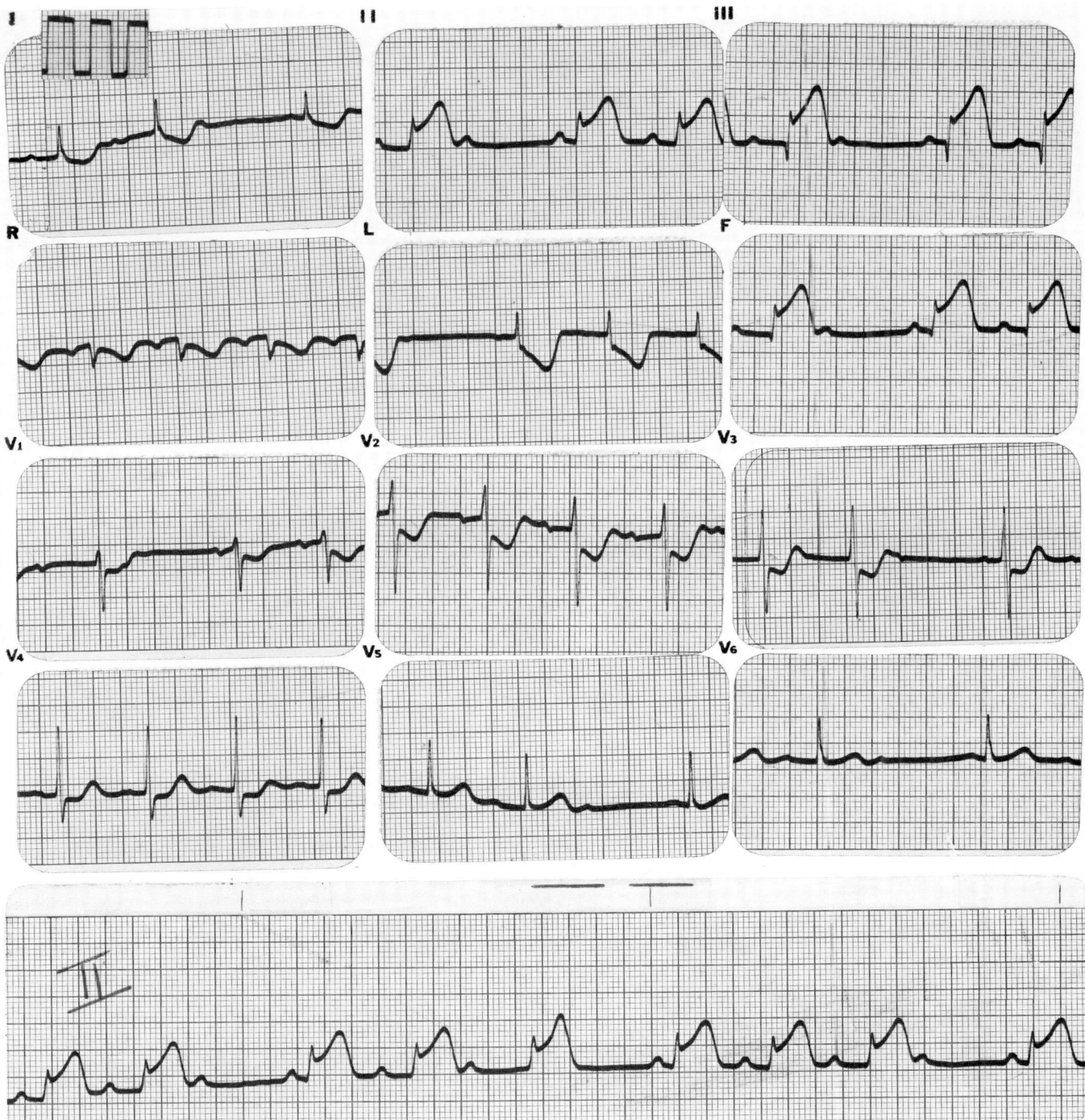

Figure 4-14.

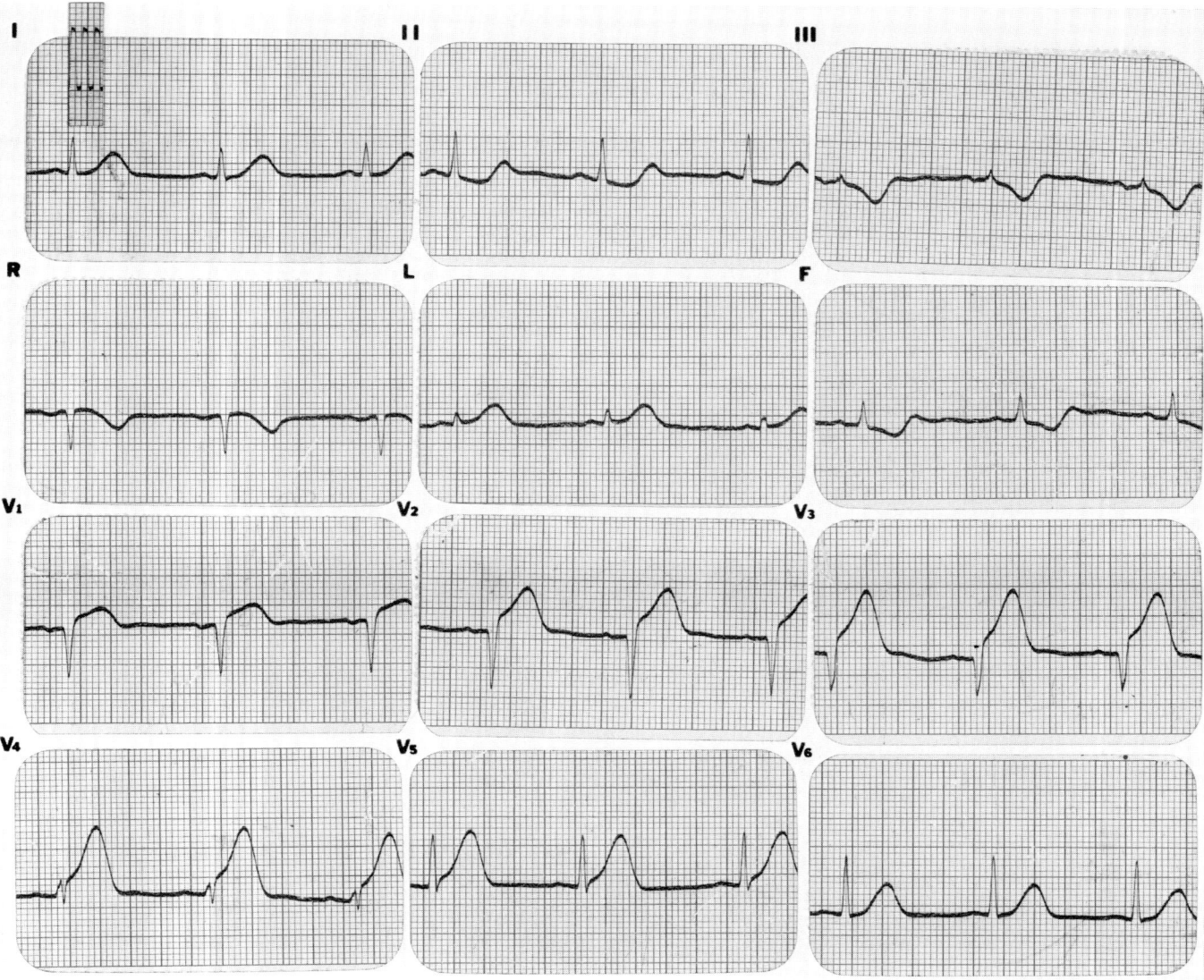

Figure 4-15A.

elevations in leads II, III and F they are diagnostic of early, acute inferior infarction. The ST segment depressions in leads I, L and V_1 to V_4 do not indicate ischemia. These are reciprocal depressions and are seen in leads on the opposite side of the heart from the ST elevations. The odds are against this patient's dying of pump failure. As far as a pacemaker is concerned, we see no ectopic beats on this tracing, and the average ventricular rate is just under 70 per minute; so there is no need to pace at the present time. Even if complete heart block or AV dissociation were to follow, with an acute inferior infarction the patient would probably have a junctional rhythm stable enough to tide him over until normal conduction returned, and so would probably not need a pacemaker.

Figure 4-15*A* shows normal sinus rhythm with a normal PR interval and narrow QRS complexes without abnormal axis deviation, so there is no conduction abnormality. There are QS complexes in

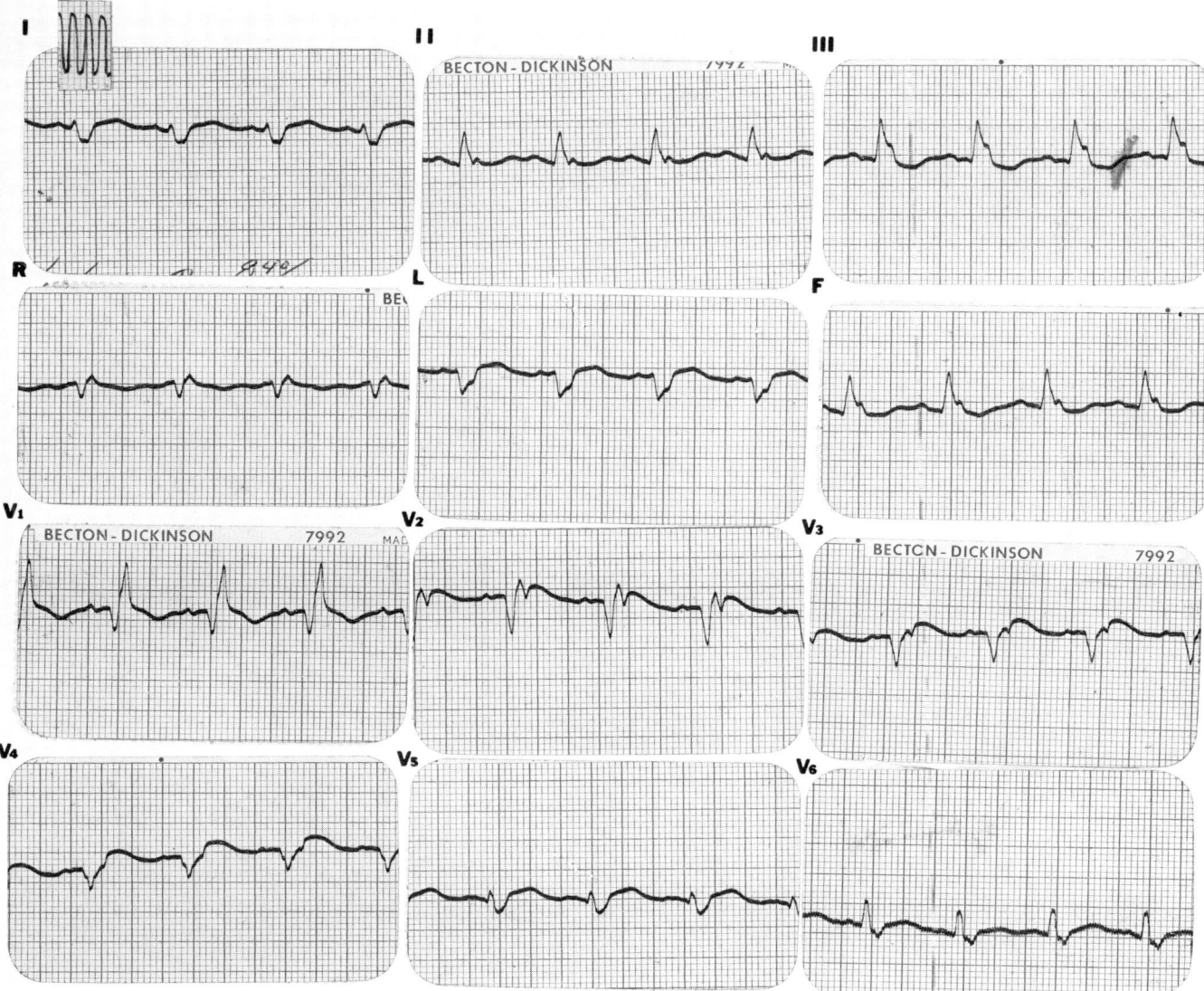

Figure 4-15B (taken 1 day after 4-15A).

V_{1-3} and a very small R wave in V_4. ST segment elevations are present in leads V_{1-4} and the T waves are tall and upright in V_{1-3}, indicating an early, acute anteroseptal infarction. The ST segment depressions in leads II, III and F are the reciprocal changes expected in acute, transmural infarction.

Figure 4-15B is from the same patient one day later. Pathologic Q waves are now present in V_{1-5}, so the infarction is even larger than it appeared in Figure 4-15A; it is an extensive anterior infarction. There are other changes, too. The QRS complexes have widened to .14 second with a QR in V_1 and a wide S wave in V_6, indicating right bundle branch block. Abnormal right axis deviation as well as small Q waves in II, III and F are now present; since we don't have evidence for a lateral wall infarction, the axis shift must have been caused by left posterior hemiblock. Therefore, this patient has an acute, extensive anterior infarction with a new bifascicular block. A temporary pacemaker should be placed because of the high likelihood of sudden

114 / Basic Electrocardiography Handbook

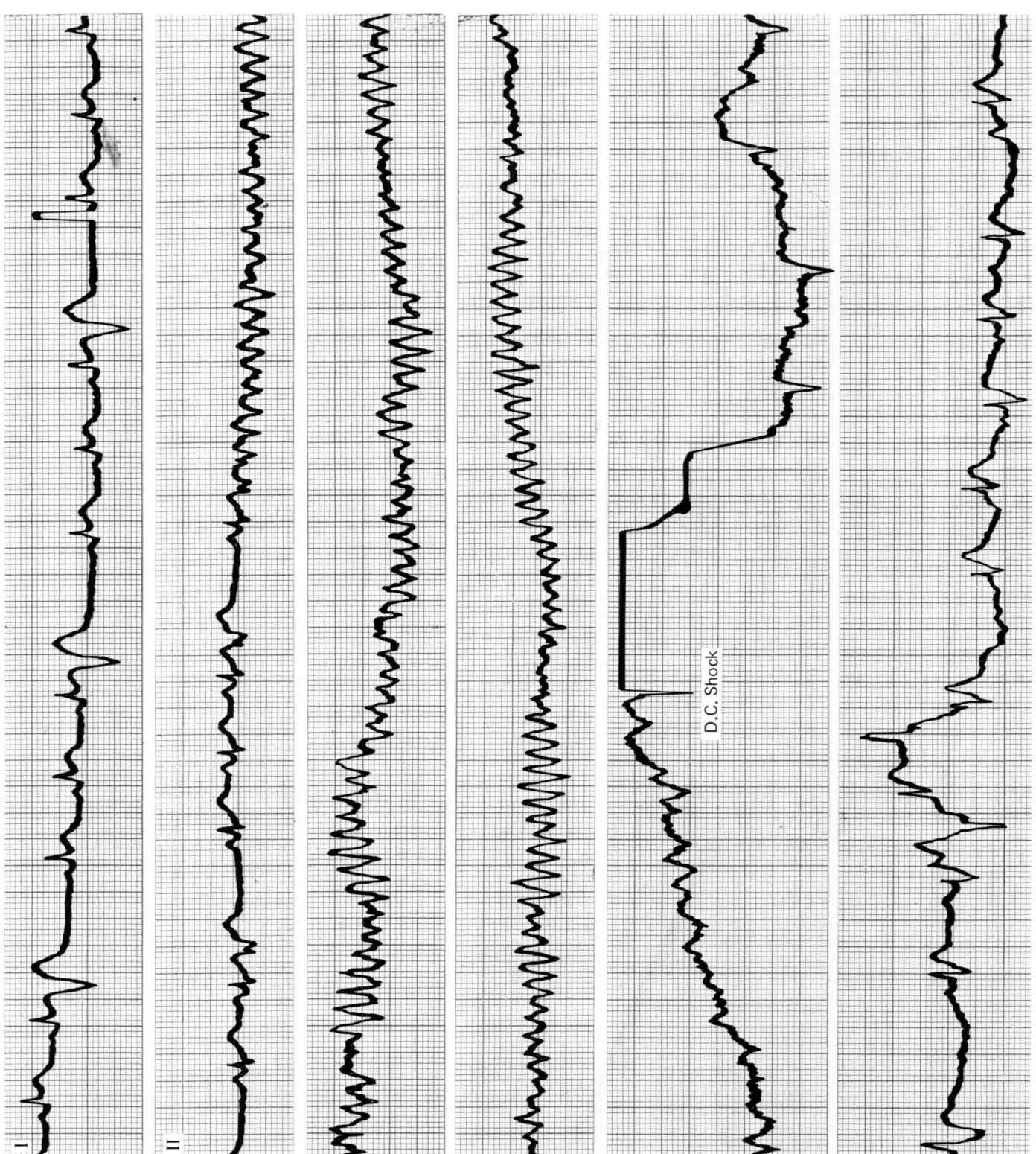

Figure 4-16.

progression to complete heart block. Unfortunately, the pacemaker may not be enough to save this patient; for an extensive anterior infarction complicated by bifascicular block is a very large infarction, and the chances of death in pump failure are great.

ARRHYTHMIAS IN ACUTE MYOCARDIAL INFARCTION

Any cardiac arrhythmia may complicate acute myocardial infarction. However, this discussion will be limited to those that are either especially dangerous or especially common, including ventricular tachycardia and fibrillation, ventricular premature beats, accelerated idioventricular rhythm and bradycardias. For all arrhythmias in acute infarction, the diagnostic criteria are the same as in any other kind of heart disease; so they are identified by the characteristics described in Chapter 3.

Unlike conduction disturbances, which usually become most severe hours to days after the onset of acute infarction, certain arrhythmias often appear very early. Indeed, ventricular fibrillation, the most frequent cause of early death after acute infarction, is most likely to occur in the first hour, and becomes progressively less common thereafter. That is why many patients with acute myocardial infarction die before reaching the hospital. In other words, the earlier a patient is seen after the onset of acute infarction, the greater the risk is that ventricular fibrillation will develop. Therefore, any patient who arrives in an emergency room complaining of chest pain should be immediately placed on a monitor with a defibrillator nearby. Such a patient should not be sent to a waiting room and told to "wait his turn" away from medical and nursing personnel. Likewise, after a decision has been made to admit such a patient, he should not be sent to various locations in the hospital like the admitting office or the X-ray department, but rather should be transported directly to the intensive care unit—ideally, accompanied by a portable monitor/defibrillator unit.

Figure 4-16 is the beginning of an electrocardiogram recorded in an emergency room on a patient who arrived after experiencing less than one hour of chest pain. Lead I and the first part of Lead II show sinus rhythm and frequent ventricular premature beats occurring during the vulnerable period. Finally, one of the premature beats causes ventricular fibrillation. Fortunately, a prompt direct current electric shock terminated the arrhythmia, and he is still alive and active six years later.

Because of the observation that many cases of ventricular fibrillation are preceded by other, less serious ventricular arrhythmias,

Table 4-2. "Warning Arrhythmias"

1. More than 5 VPB per minute
2. Multifocal VPB (any number)
3. VPB falling on the preceding T wave ("R on T phenomenon")
4. VPB in salvos
5. Ventricular tachycardia, no matter how brief

116 / Basic Electrocardiography Handbook

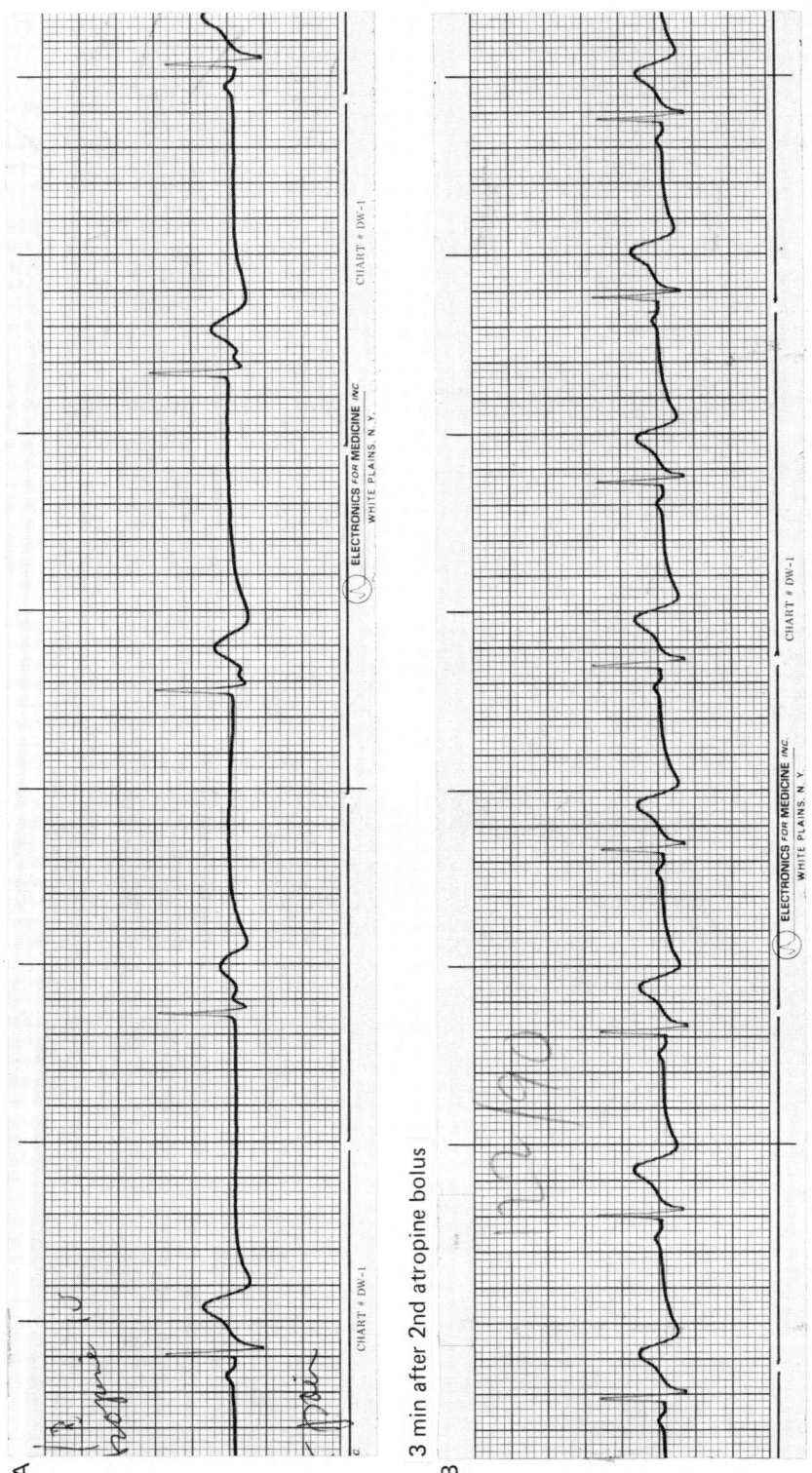

3 min after 2nd atropine bolus

Figure 4-17.

it has become standard practice to administer medication, usually intravenous lidocaine (Xylocaine), in order to prevent ventricular fibrillation when any of the so-called warning arrhythmias appears in a patient with acute myocardial infarction (Table 4-2). Use of lidocaine is reasonably safe in these circumstances *provided that the sinus rate exceeds 60 per minute*—if it is slower, the drug may cause further slowing and actually increase rather than decrease the numbers of ventricular premature beats. Without doubt, ventricular fibrillation is prevented in many cases by prompt treatment of these arrhythmias. However, we now know that sometimes, especially in very early infarction, the first ventricular premature beat starts ventricular fibrillation, and in other cases the warning beats only precede ventricular fibrillation by 10 or 20 seconds—insufficient time for any drug to be prepared, be injected, circulate in the body and have a beneficial effect. To avoid this problem, we may someday see all patients with suspected or proven acute myocardial infarction being treated with drugs to prevent ventricular fibrillation as well as other complications. At present, however, this type of treatment is experimental.

Accelerated idioventricular rhythm is one of the most common arrhythmias in acute infarction, but it is not a dangerous rhythm—in fact, it usually causes no problems at all unless it is confused with ventricular tachycardia. Normal sinus rhythm soon returns even if nothing is done, so usually no treatment is required.

Bradycardias constitute a very important group of arrhythmias in acute myocardial infarction, especially inferior infarction and particularly in the first minutes to hours. Any rhythm with a heart rate under 60 is a bradycardia. (See list in Table 4-3.)

Although bradycardias are sometimes well tolerated by patients with acute myocardial infarction, frequently bradycardias lead to a fall in cardiac output or other more serious arrhythmias, particularly when they are slower than 50 per minute. When cardiac output is diminished by a bradycardia, the usual result is low blood pressure. Inadequate blood supply to the brain causes confusion or drowsiness. Other organs such as the kidneys, liver and intestines may also malfunction until the cardiac output is increased by correction of the bradycardia. Figure 4-17*A* is a monitor lead rhythm strip from a patient with an acute inferior infarction. It shows a severe sinus bradycardia and a slow junctional escape rhythm at 35 per minute. Consequently, the patient's blood pressure was very low (60 systolic, diastolic undetectable). After treatment with atropine (strip *B*), the sinus rate accelerated to 58 per minute. Although this rhythm is

Table 4-3. Bradycardias

1. Sinus bradycardia
2. Sinus arrest or sinoatrial block
3. Junctional rhythm
4. Idioventricular rhythm
5. Second and third degree AV block
6. Atrial fibrillation with slow ventricular response

still a bradycardia, the improvement in the heart rate was enough to raise the blood pressure to 120/90, and no further treatment was required.

When ventricular arrhythmias complicate bradycardias, the drugs that ordinarily control ventricular arrhythmias are usually ineffective and frequently aggravate the situation by making the bradycardia slower still. Drugs such as lidocaine, procaineamide (Pronestyl), quinidine, digitalis and propanolol (Inderal) are dangerous to use in the presence of a bradycardia. However, acceleration of the heart rate by drugs (atropine, isoproterenol) or a pacemaker if the drugs fail often abolishes the ventricular ectopic rhythm as the bradycardia is corrected.

Chapter 5
Electrocardiographic Diagnosis in Other Diseases

ACUTE PERICARDITIS

Myocardial ischemia and infarction are by no means the only causes of chest pain lasting a half hour or more. There are numerous other causes—some minor, others potentially serious. One that is frequently confused with acute myocardial infarction is acute pericarditis, an inflammation of the pericardium. Since the pain of pericarditis originates from the heart, it may be felt in the same area as the pain of infarction. However, the pain of pericarditis is almost always *pleuritic* (increased by inhaling), while the pain of myocardial ischemia or infarction is not. The pleuritic character of pericarditis pain makes it easy to distinguish the two conditions, even when pericarditis occurs in a patient with acute myocardial infarction. Indeed, many patients have pericarditis two to four days after acute myocardial infarction as part of the healing process. A smaller number have pericarditis several weeks later, probably because of an unusual type of allergic reaction brought on by the infarction. Since pericarditis does not significantly affect the myocardium, and since it does not lead to the potentially fatal arrhythmias and conduction disorders of myocardial infarction, intensive care is not required, and the patient can be assured that he is not undergoing further heart damage. The typical pain is sometimes the only indication that pericarditis is present, but the electrocardiogram is often confirmatory. In acute pericarditis, ST segments are usually elevated in all leads except AVR and sometimes V_1, where they may be normal or depressed.

Figure 5-1 shows the typical electrocardiographic picture of acute pericarditis. ST segment elevations with increased T wave amplitude are obviously present in leads I and V_{2-6}. These look just like the changes of acute myocardial infarction (Figure 4-1A, Chapter 4) except that instead of reciprocal ST depressions in the inferior leads,

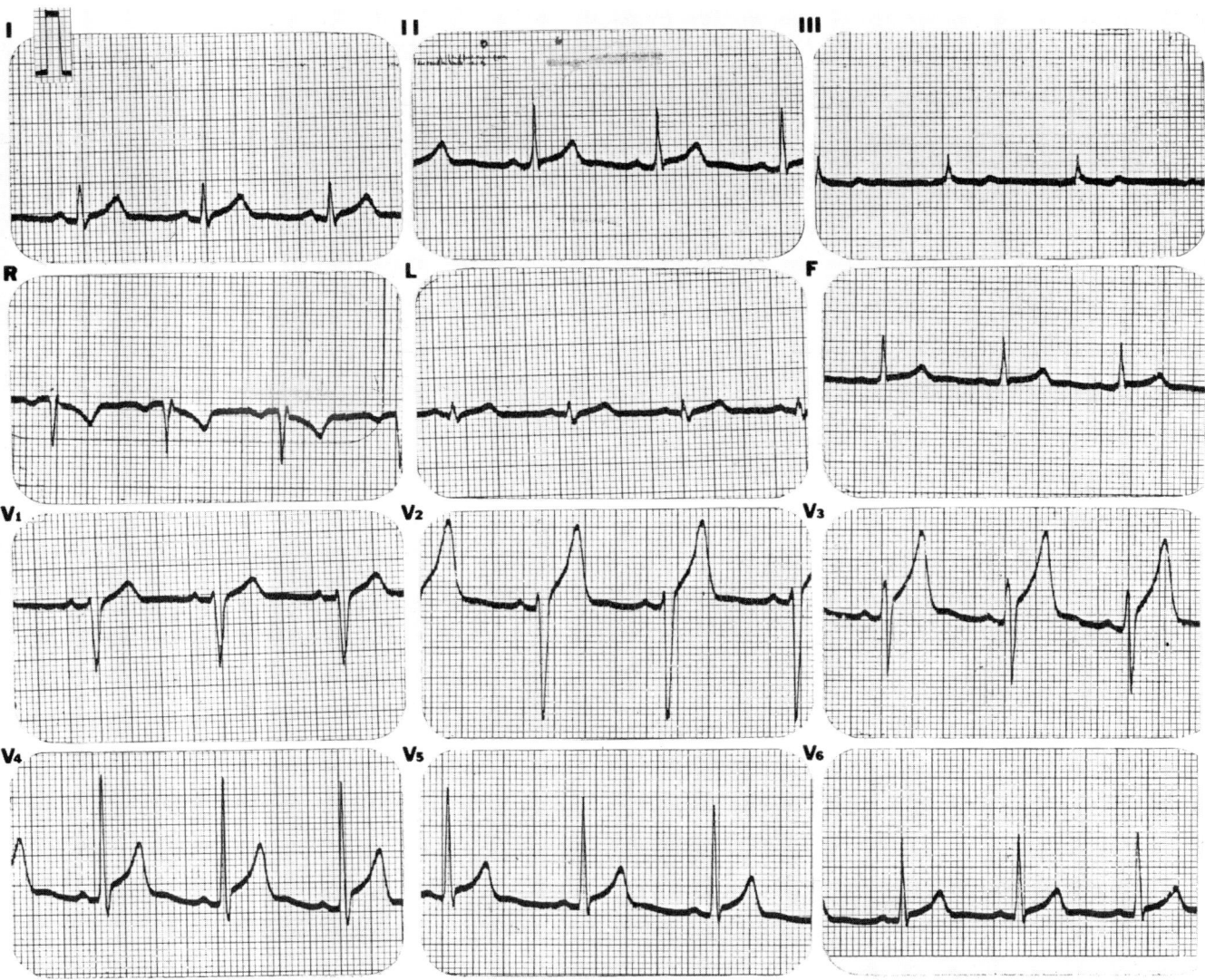

Figure 5-1.

there are also ST elevations in leads II, III and F as well as L and V_1. Only lead R has depressed ST segments. Later on in the course of acute pericarditis the ST segments return to normal, and the T waves may become inverted. Figure 5-2, recorded two days after Figure 5-1, shows that the ST segments are not as elevated, and the T wave amplitude has diminished in every lead except R. In some leads (V_{2-5}) the T waves have become inverted.

The electrocardiogram is less helpful in diagnosing acute pericarditis following acute myocardial infarction than when the pericarditis affects a previously normal heart. However, in some cases the electrocardiogram will show the typical generalized ST segment elevations, and the previous reciprocal depressions will disappear. Such a case is shown in Figures 5-3, 5-4 and 5-5.

Figure 5-3 shows the typical changes of early, acute extensive anterior myocardial infarction: elevation of the ST segments and

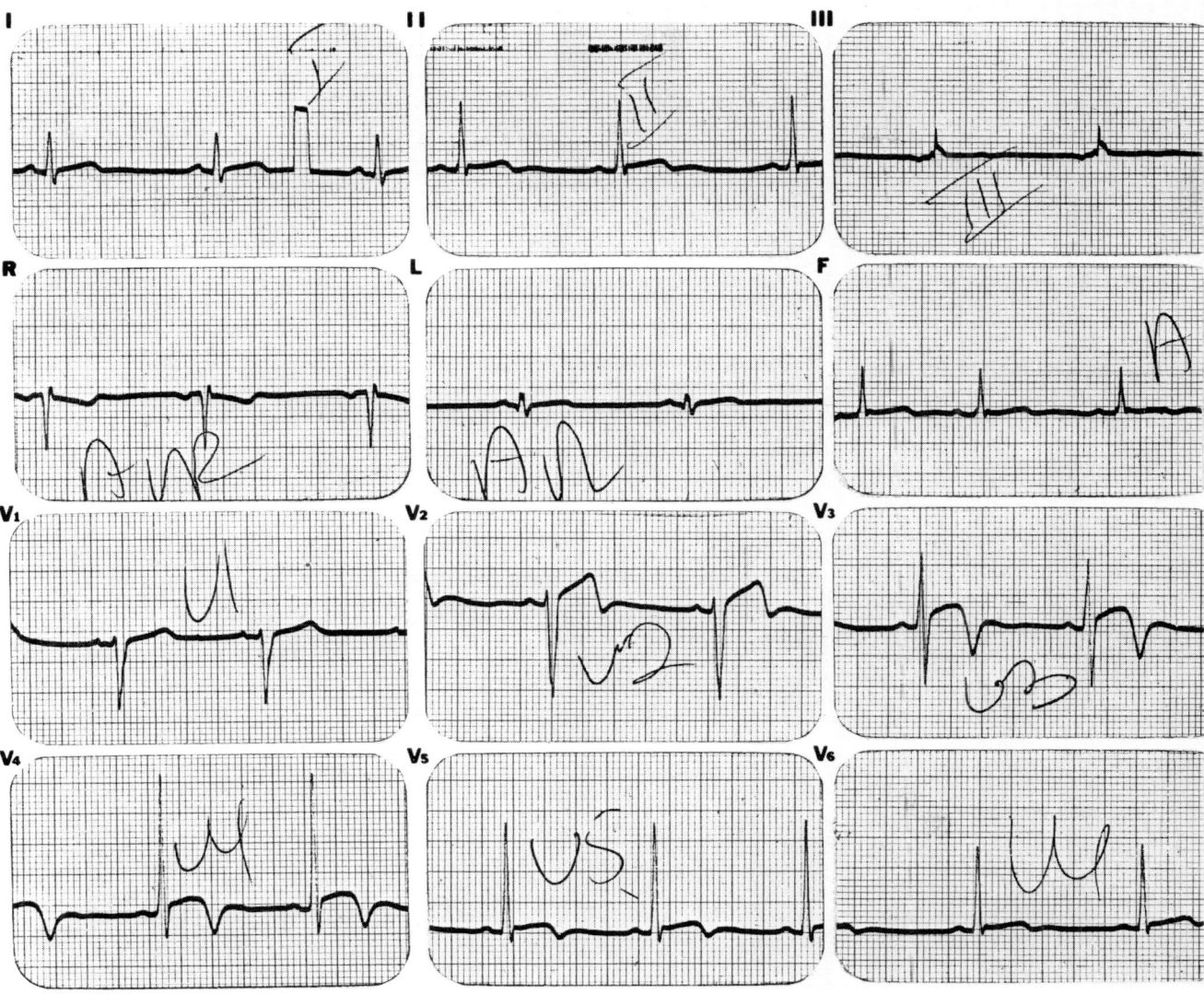

Figure 5-2.

increased T wave amplitude in leads I and V_{1-5}, and slight reciprocal ST segment depressions in leads III and F. Three days later (Figure 5-4) the patient developed the typical pleuritic chest pain of pericarditis. In addition to new pathological Q waves in leads V_{1-3}, and diminution of the height of the T waves in leads V_{1-4}, there are now ST segment elevations in all leads except R. Several days later (Figure 5-5) the changes of acute pericarditis are no longer present, and the electrocardiogram only shows the changes of recent extensive anterior infarction.

An unusual, but striking, electrocardiographic pattern is seen in some cases of pericarditis with *effusion* (fluid collection). This pattern is called *electrical alternans*, since every other QRS complex looks different. Electrical alternans probably occurs because the heart is not firmly supported when a large pericardial effusion is present. Instead, the heart is suspended in the fluid-filled pericardial

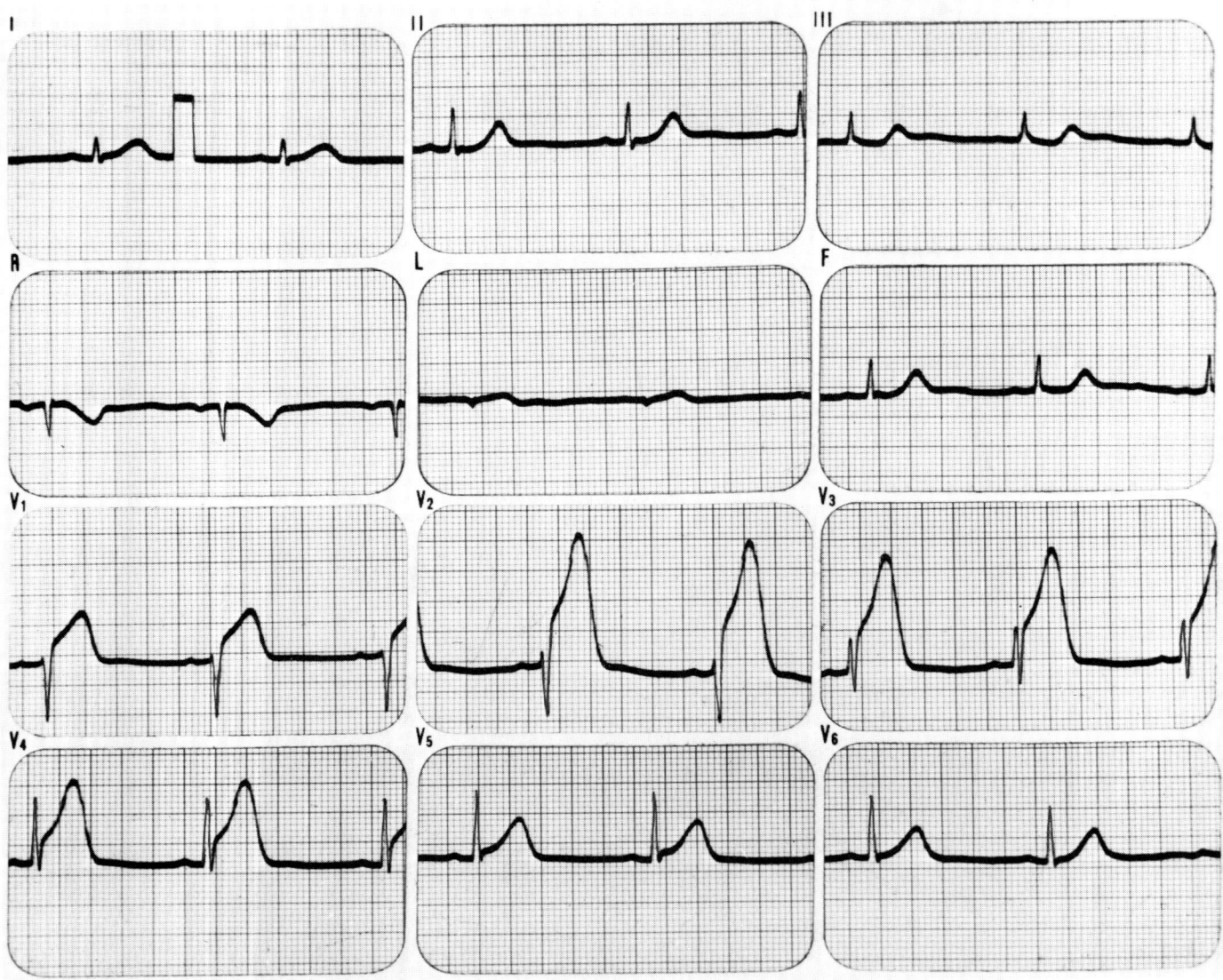

Figure 5-3.

sac, and so rocks back and forth with each succeeding beat. Electrical alternans is said to be especially common when pericarditis with effusion is caused by metastatic cancer deposits in the pericardium. Figure 5-6 is an example of electrical alternans recorded from a patient with metastatic breast cancer. The alternating QRS complexes are most obvious in leads III, V_1, V_3, V_4 and V_5, but close inspection shows electrical alternans in every lead.

PULMONARY EMBOLISM

Embolism is the sudden blocking of an artery by material (*embolus;* plural, *emboli*) that has traveled through the bloodstream. Emboli to the pulmonary arteries are most often clots (thromboemboli) which originate elsewhere in the body, but they may be fat (especially

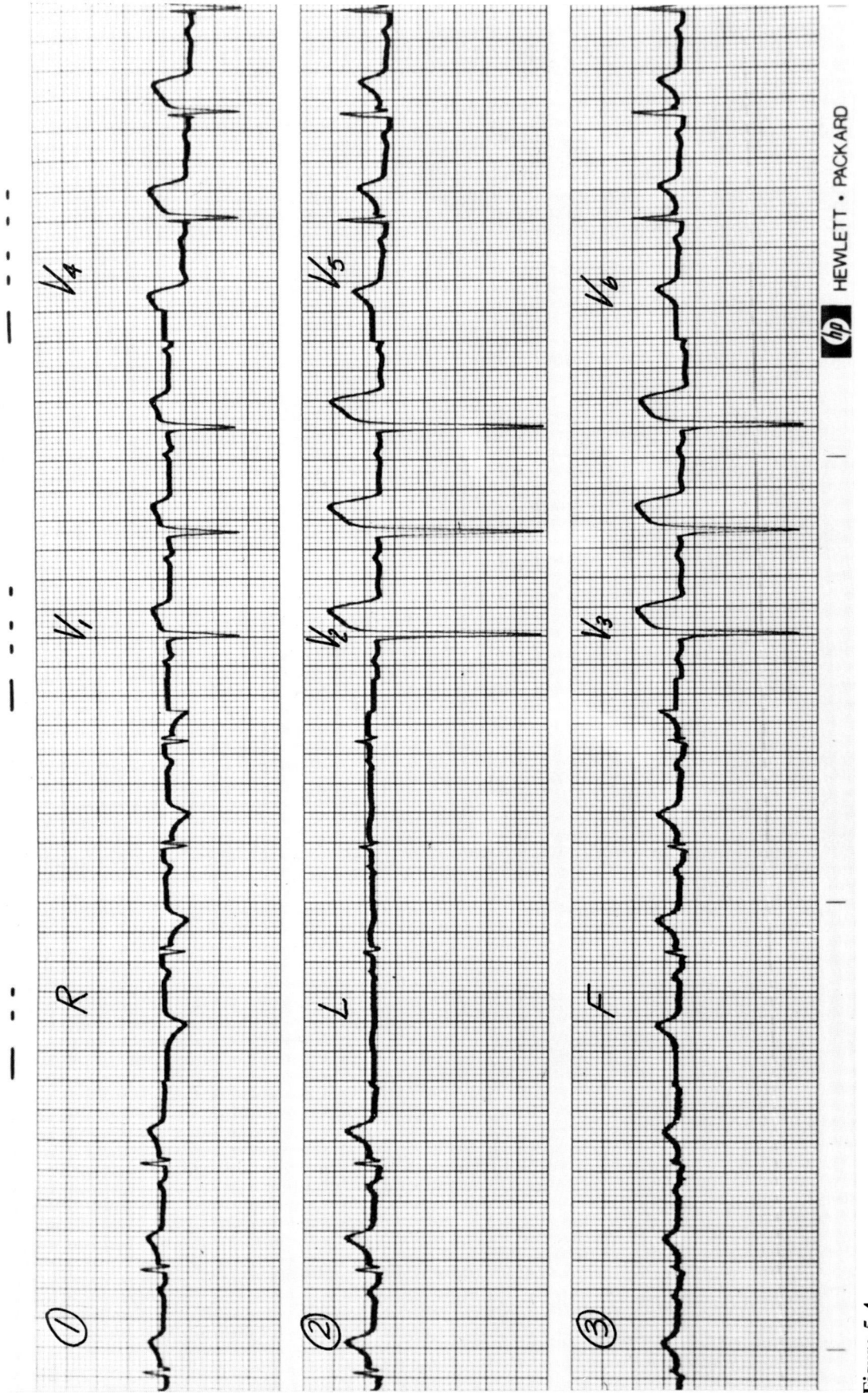

Figure 5-4.

124 / **Basic Electrocardiography Handbook**

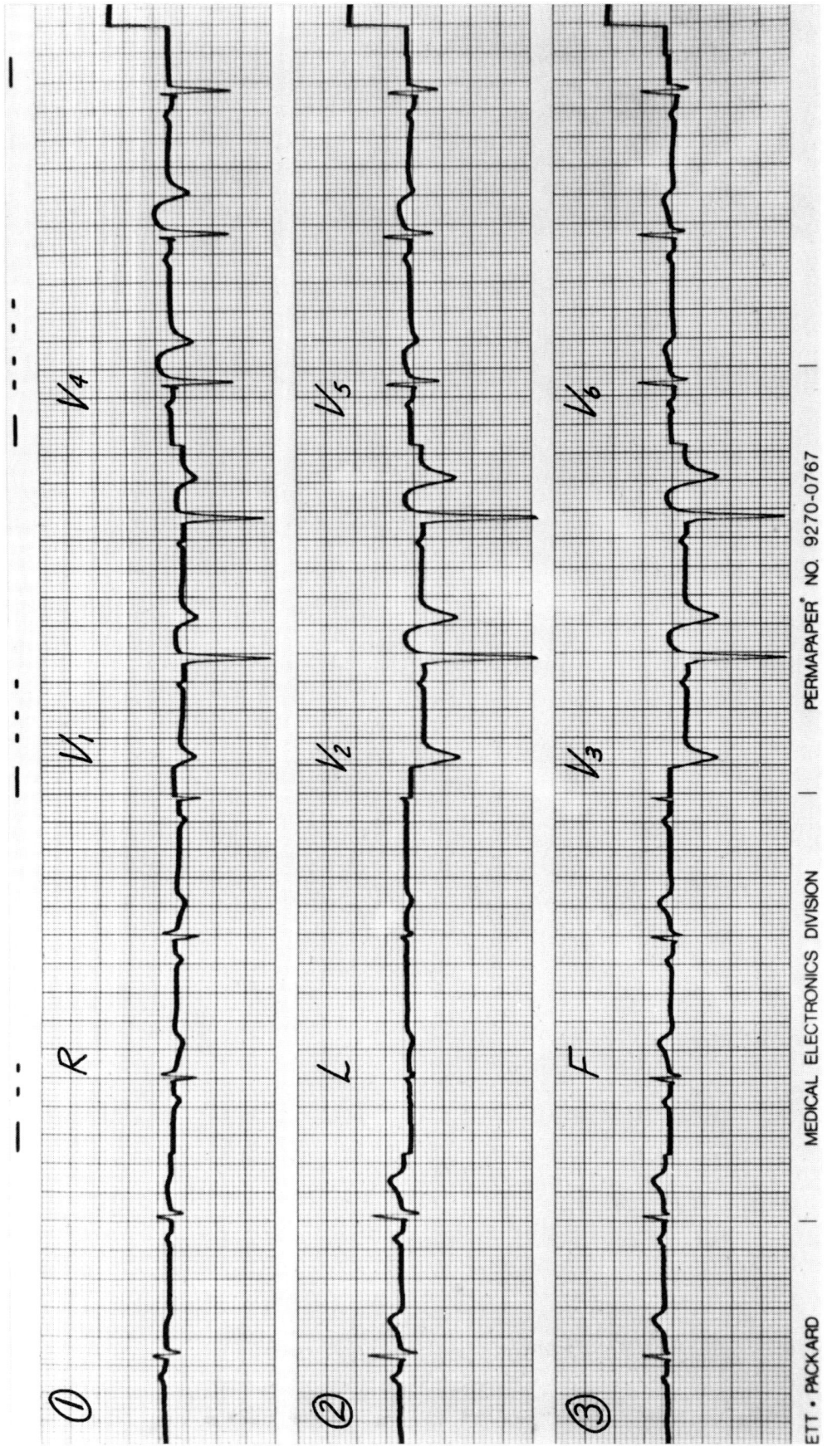

Figure 5-5.

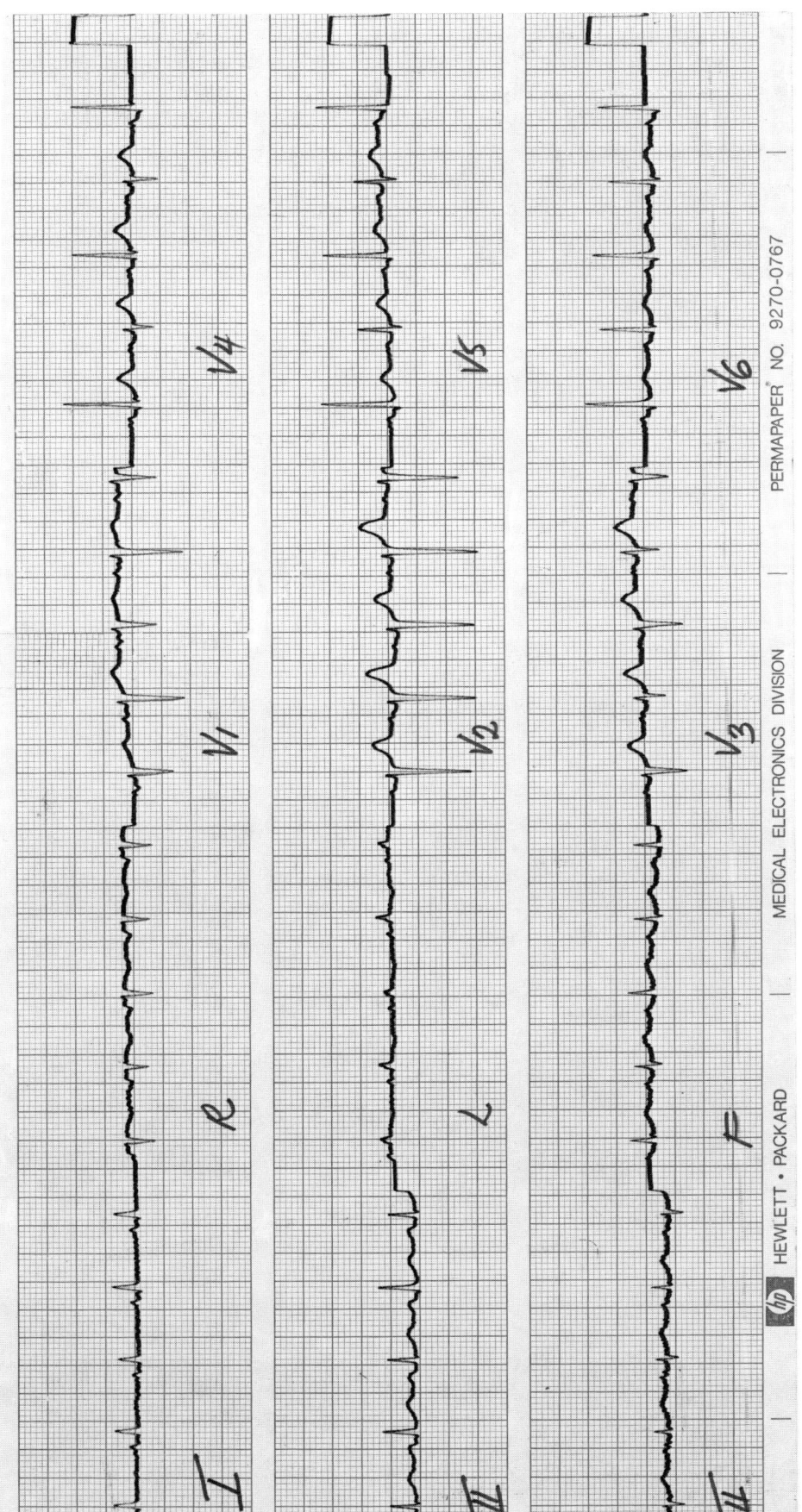

Figure 5-6.

within 48 hours of a major fracture), amniotic (tissues related to pregnancy that may be forced into the mother's bloodstream during complicated deliveries) or other material. Large pulmonary emboli may result in chest pain; but often the pain is minimal and sudden shortness of breath, rapid breathing, tachycardia, fall in blood pressure or syncope are the initial signs. Unfortunately, in some cases the electrocardiogram remains normal, and in many others the only abnormalities are sinus tachycardia and nonspecific ST segment and/or T abnormalities. However, the diagnosis should be strongly considered when sudden shortness of breath or any of the other symptoms is accompanied by one or more of the following:

1. New incomplete or complete right bundle branch block
2. Sudden right axis deviation
3. ST segment depressions and T wave inversions confined to the right chest leads (V_1, V_2 and V_3)
4. New S waves in leads I and V_6 with a Q wave and T inversion in III

HYPERKALEMIA

Hyperkalemia (too much potassium in the blood) and the other disorders to be discussed in this chapter do not cause chest pain but may cause serious or even fatal arrhythmias if they are not recognized and treated appropriately. Often the diagnosis can only be made by electrocardiogram or blood tests, since the patient may have no symptoms at all

The body can eliminate potassium only through the kidneys, so hyperkalemia is always a danger in cases of kidney failure, particularly when urine output is small or absent. Hyperkalemia can also be caused by diuretics (spironolactone [Aldactone] and triamterene [Dyrenium]) that interfere with the kidneys' ability to excrete potassium.

High concentrations of potassium in the blood depress electrical and mechanical functions of the heart, so the end result of untreated hyperkalemia is death in asystole. Fortunately, elevated but sublethal concentrations of potassium usually cause easily recognizable changes in the electrocardiogram

Figure 5-8 shows the electrocardiogram of a patient with mild hyperkalemia, to compare with the same patient's electrocardiogram (Figure 5-7) recorded when the serum potassium content was normal. The only difference is a symmetrical increase in the height of the T waves in all leads, so-called peaking of the T waves. The symmetry of the T waves is important, because tall T waves that are not symmetrical usually do signify hyperkalemia.

In more severe hyperkalemia, as illustrated by another patient in Figure 5-9, depression of intraatrial conduction causes the P waves to become smaller or disappear altogether. Depression of intraventricular conduction causes the QRS complexes to widen, and frequently develop axis shifts because of fascicular block.

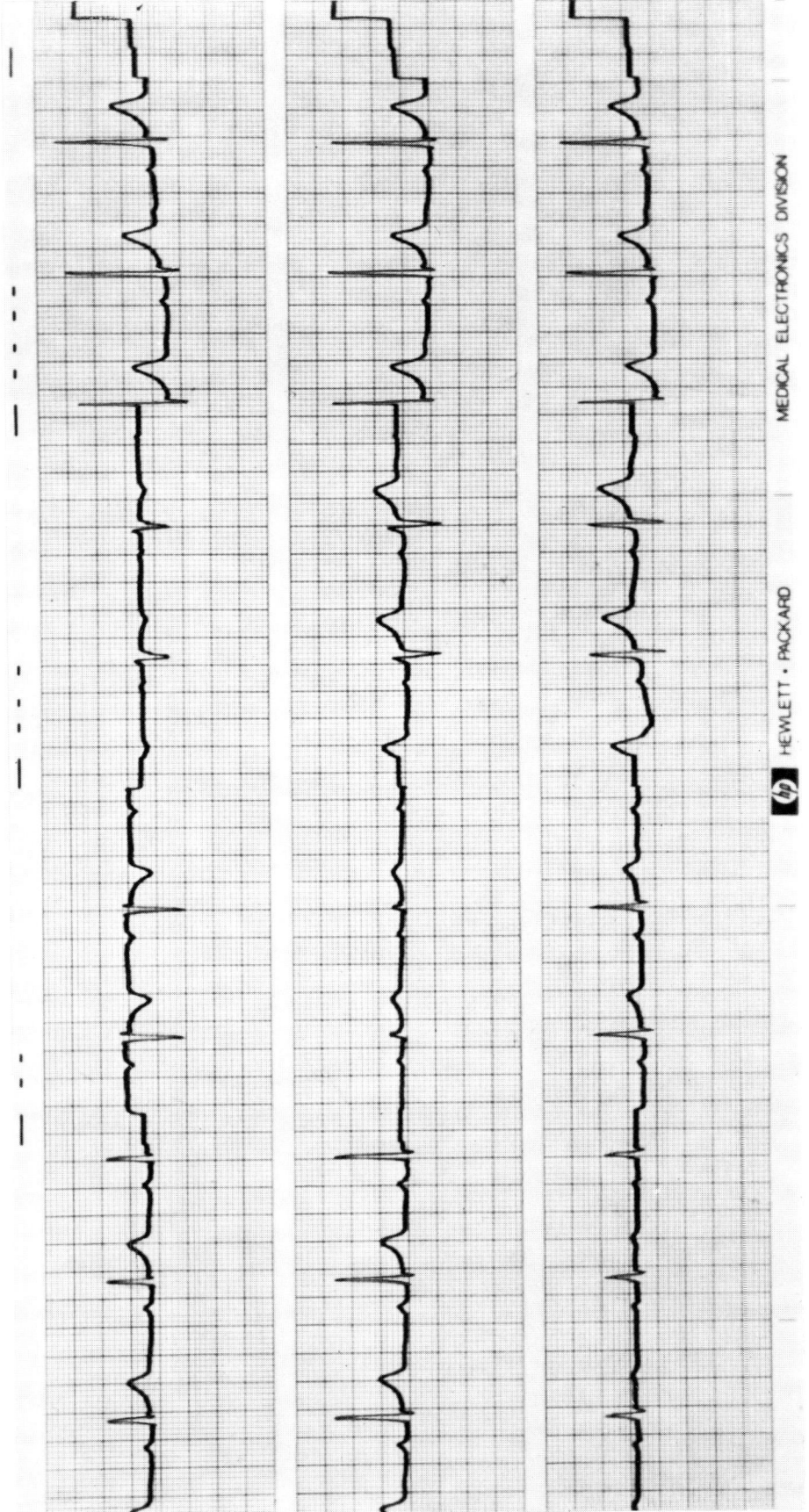

Figure 5-7.

128 / Basic Electrocardiography Handbook

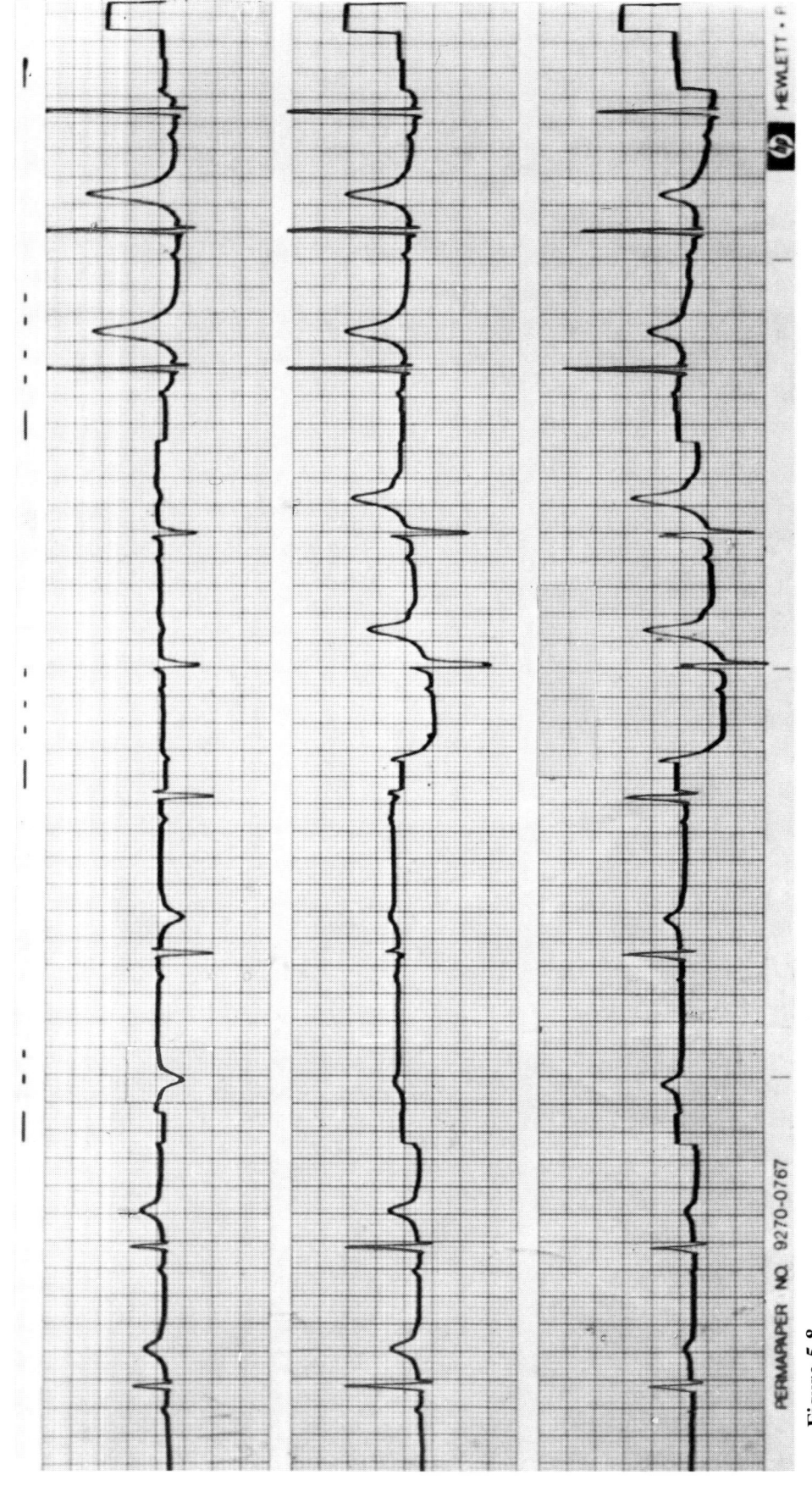

Figure 5-8.

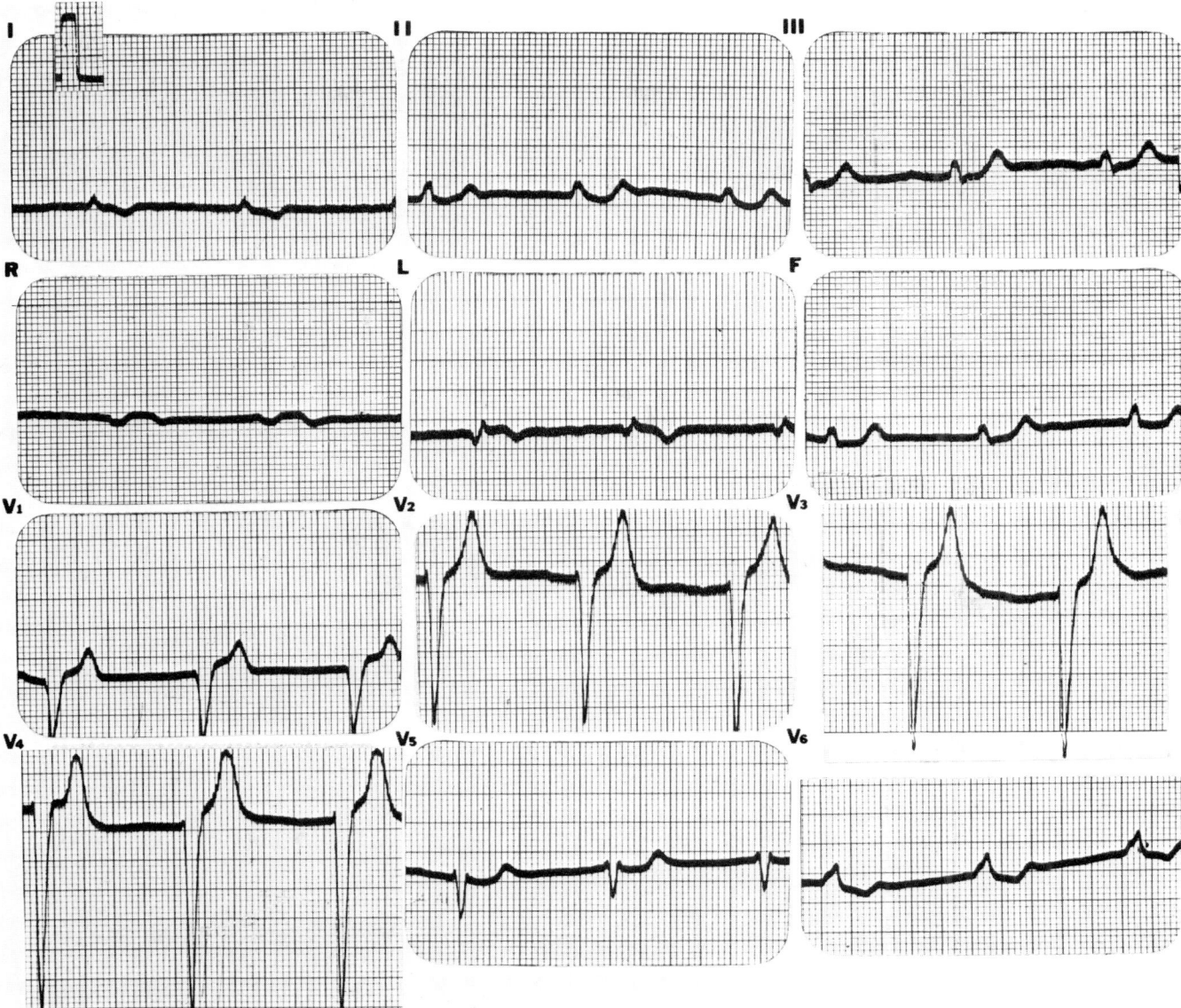

Figure 5-9.

In the most extreme cases of hyperkalemia, like the one shown in Figure 5-10, bizarre, wide QRS complexes merge with the ST segment and T wave, so that it is hard to tell where one ends and the other begins. Changes in QRS configuration in hyperkalemia do not necessarily represent ectopic beats—often the changes reflect changing intraventricular conduction disturbances. Fortunately, even the most severe cases of hyperkalemia can be temporarily stabilized within minutes by sodium bicarbonate injected intravenously, and afterwards other methods can be used to eliminate the excess potassium. The electrocardiogram in Figure 5-11 was recorded from the same patient as Figure 5-10, immediately after the intravenous injection of sodium bicarbonate. Notice the remarkable improvement in the appearance of the QRS complexes.

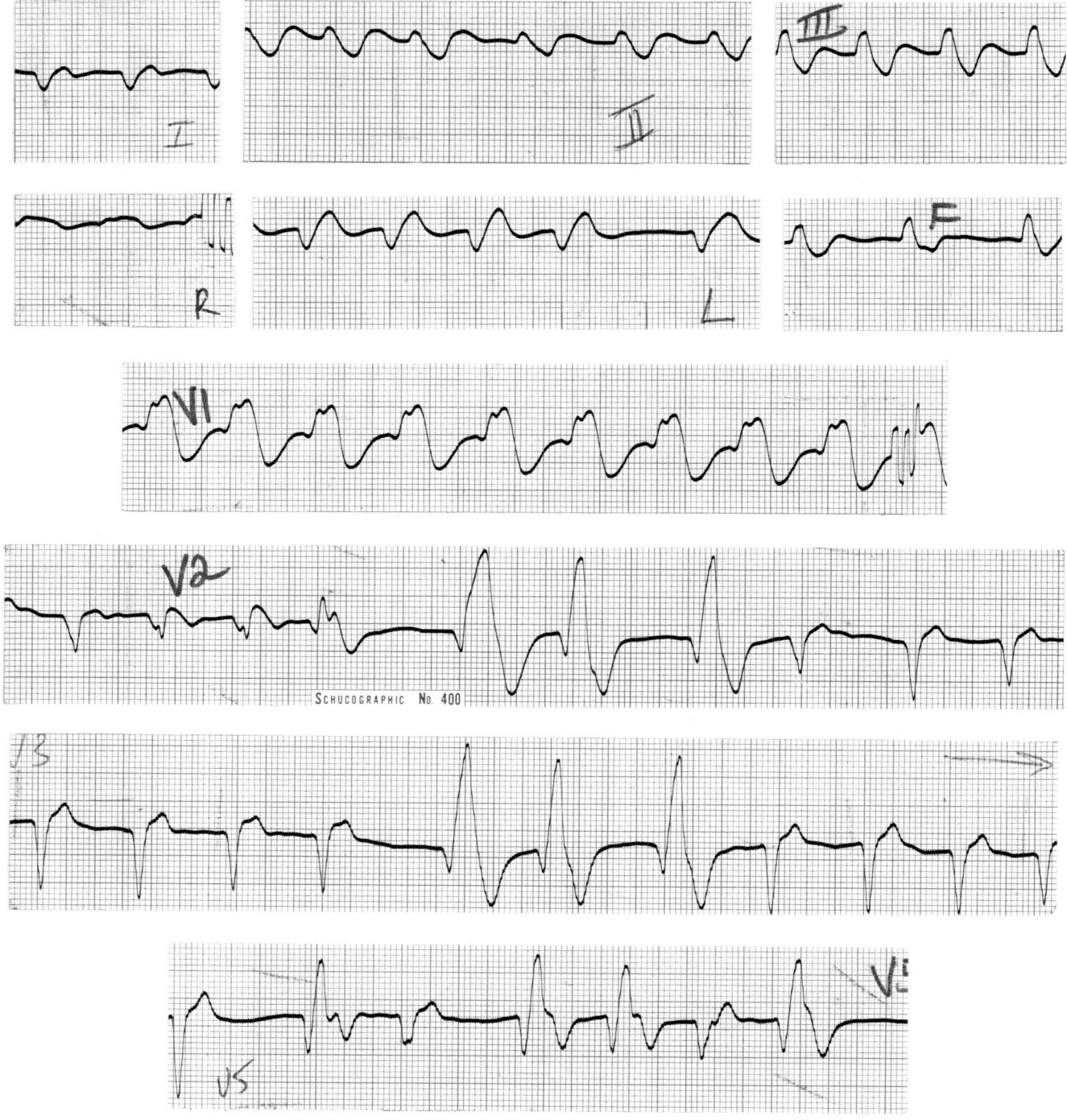

Figure 5-10.

HYPOKALEMIA

Hypokalemia (too little potassium in the blood) may result from excess loss through the kidneys, particularly in patients treated with any diuretic other than spironolactone or triamterene, or with cortisone-type drugs, or who have uncontrolled diabetes mellitus. Potassium may also be lost from the intestinal tract by patients with severe diarrhea and those on prolonged nasogastric suction. Hypokalemia makes the heart more irritable, and may cause any of the ventricular arrhythmias seen in acute myocardial infarction, including ventricular fibrillation. Hypokalemia is dangerous by itself, but even more dangerous in patients receiving digitalis, since digitalis toxic rhythms appear at much lower digitalis concentrations in hypokalemic patients than under any other circumstance.

The characteristic electrocardiographic changes of hypokalemia are mild ST segment depression, flattening of the T wave and enlargement of the U wave, which often appears to cause a prolonged QT interval because the giant U wave is mistaken for a T wave. It is illustrated by Figure 5-12, an electrocardiogram recorded on a patient who was severely hypokalemic because of the combined effects of diuretic therapy and uncontrolled diabetes mellitus. In leads I, II and most of the other leads, the QT interval appears to be .50 second (normal being less than .40 second). On this tracing, the true T wave is visible only in lead V_1, and in that lead the QT interval is only .40 second long, proving that the "T" in the other leads is really a giant U wave.

Other Causes of Long QT or QU Intervals

A long QT or QU interval may be caused by hypokalemia, occasionally some other type of electrolyte imbalance, quinidine, procaine-amide (Pronestyl) or some drugs used for treatment of psychiatric patients, especially thioridazine (Mellaril); or it may be present from birth. Therefore, without knowing the drugs a patient is receiving, it is usually not possible to make a precise diagnosis of the cause of a long QT or QU interval from the electrocardiogram alone. Whatever the cause, however, a very long QT or QU interval indicates a serious disorder of myocardial repolarization with an increased potential for ventricular arrhythmias, including ventricular fibrillation. If such a patient shows any kind of ventricular ectopic activity, even just premature beats, it is wise to begin the same type of monitoring that one would use for a possible acute myocardial infarction, at least until the cause of abnormal repolarization is determined and preferably until the rhythm is stabilized.

PREEXCITATION

Preexcitation is a condition in which all or part of the ventricular myocardium is depolarized by sinoatrial impulses that have bypassed the AV node. Patients with preexcitation frequently suffer from recurrent supraventricular arrhythmias. Although preexcitation is

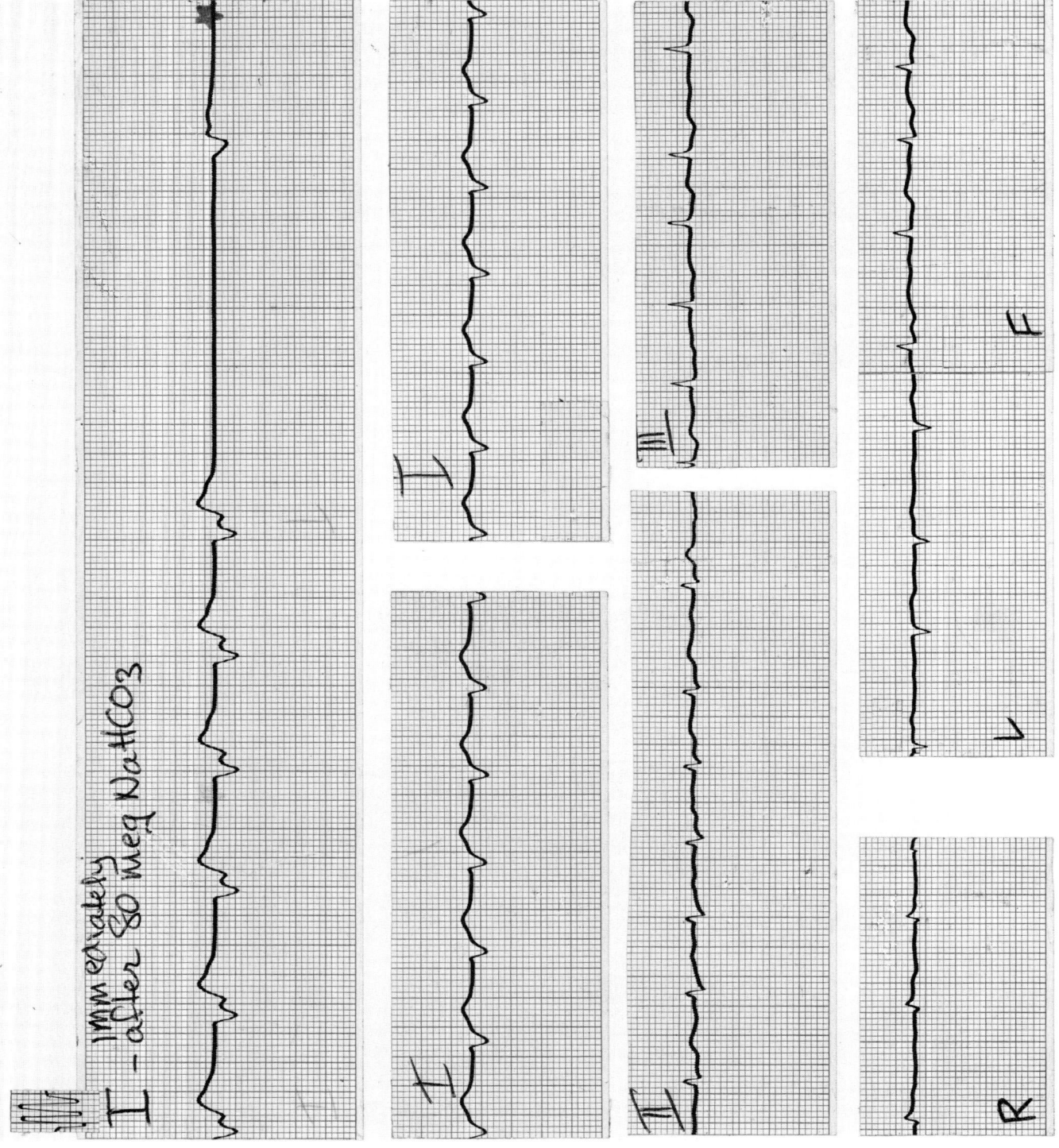

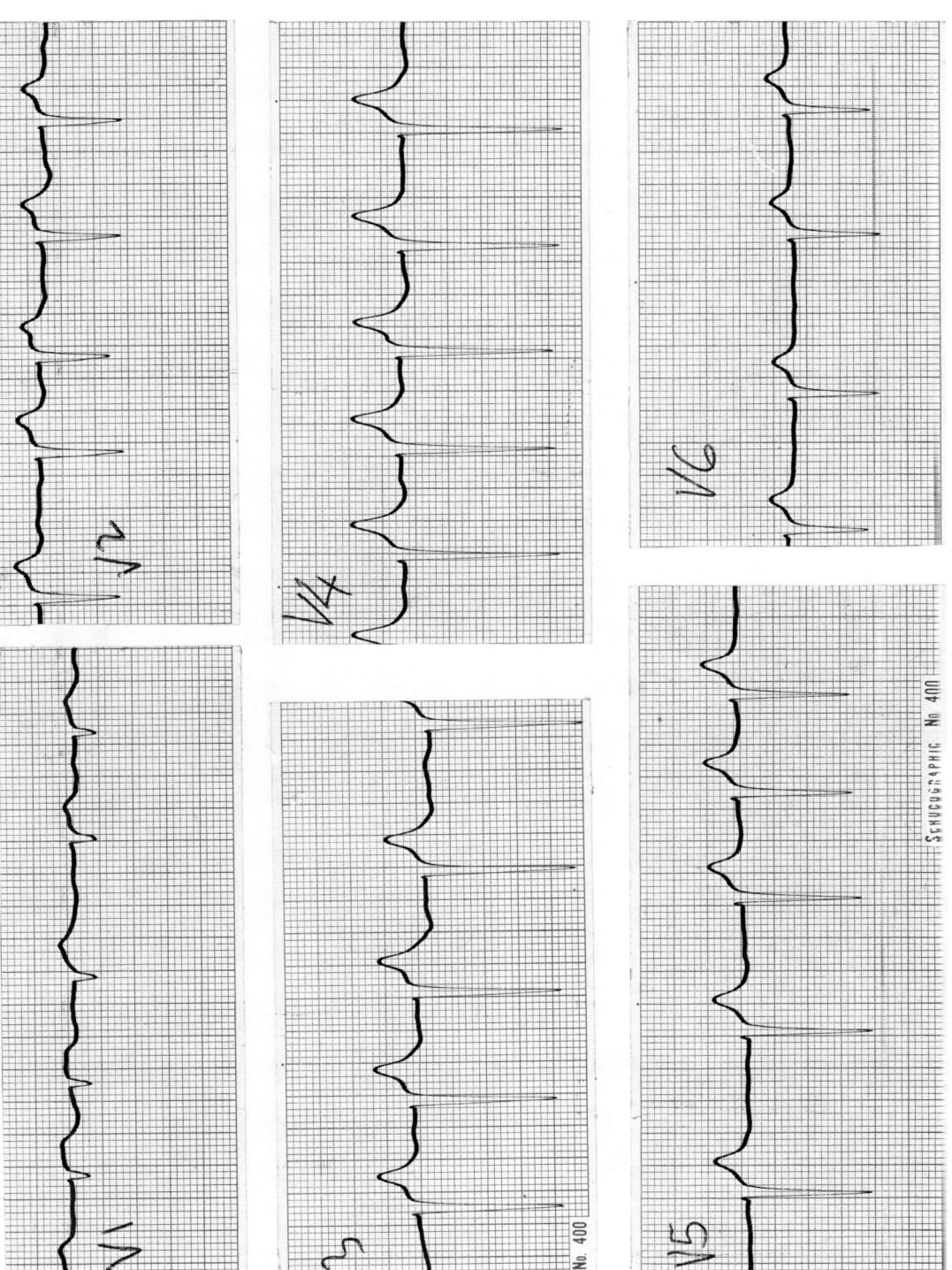

Figure 5-11.

not common, it is of particular importance to the electrocardiographer because the diagnosis is almost always made by electrocardiogram. Examination of the heart, X rays and blood tests are usually normal in patients with preexcitation.

Wolff-Parkinson-White Syndrome

Wolff-Parkinson-White syndrome is the best known form of preexcitation. Like other forms of preexcitation, it is an abnormality present from birth in which one or more accessory pathways (bypass tracts) exist, permitting sinoatrial impulses to reach the ventricles without going through the AV node. In Wolff-Parkinson-White syndrome, when a sinoatrial impulse reaches the atrial end of the bypass tract, it is conducted to the adjacent ventricular myocardium without delay because the bypass tract contains no AV nodal tissue.

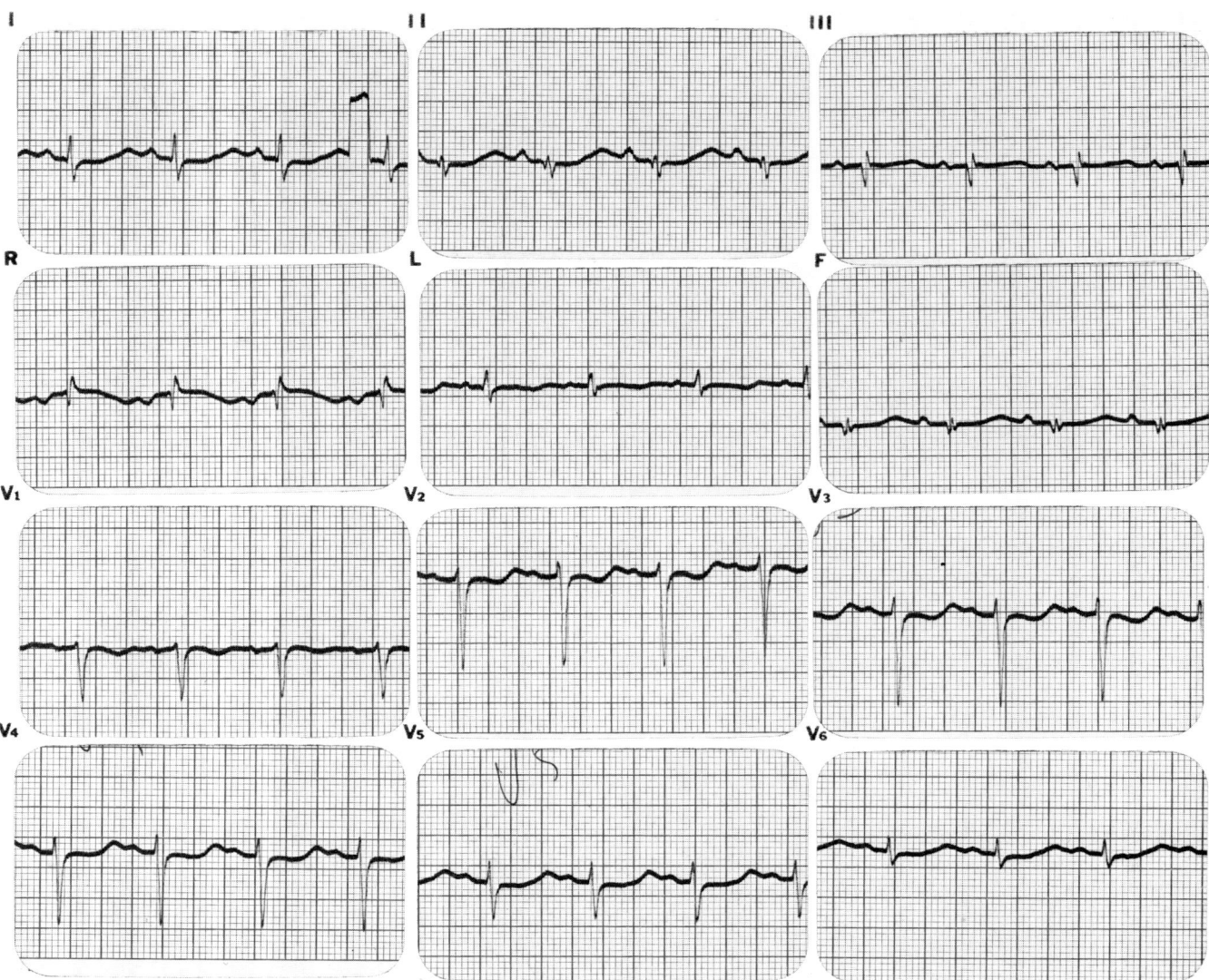

Figure 5-12.

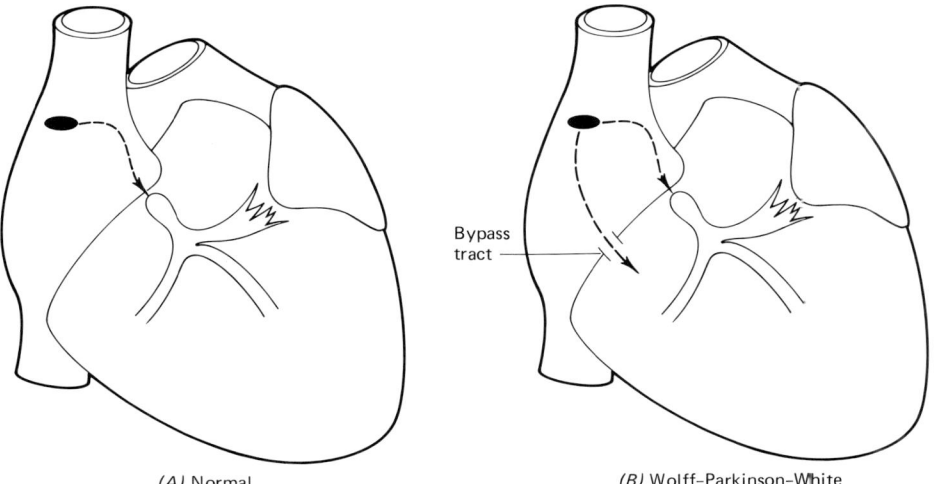

(A) Normal   *(B)* Wolff-Parkinson-White

Figure 5-13.

The ventricular myocardium around the bypass tract then depolarizes, and the impulse begins to spread slowly throughout the ventricular myocardium. Meanwhile, the same sinoatrial impulse has also passed through the AV node and, after its usual delay there, spreads in the normal rapid fashion via the His-Purkinje system throughout any part of the ventricles that have not already been depolarized via the bypass tract.

Figure 5-13 schematically contrasts the normal situation (*A*), where the sinoatrial impulse can only reach the ventricles by going through the AV node, with Wolff-Parkinson-White syndrome (*B*) where there are two pathways available.

Figure 5-14 shows how the ventricles are depolarized in Wolff-Parkinson-White syndrome. In the example shown, a bypass tract connects the right atrium and right ventricle, so that part of the right ventricle (vertical hatching) is depolarized by the impulse coming over the bypass tract, while the rest of the right ventricle and all of

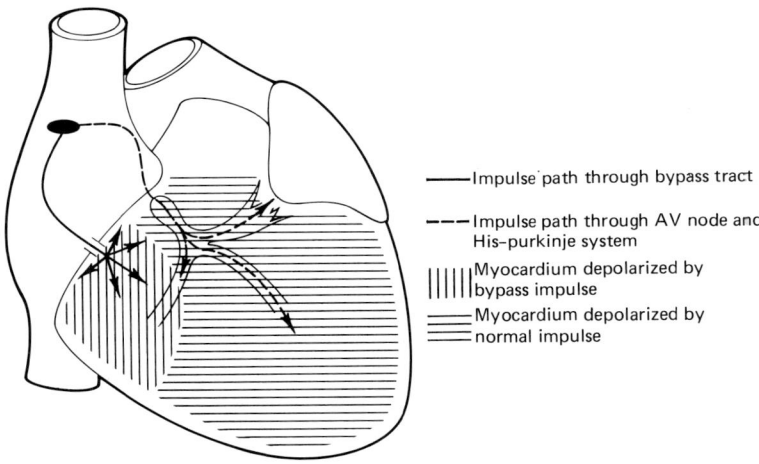

Figure 5-14.

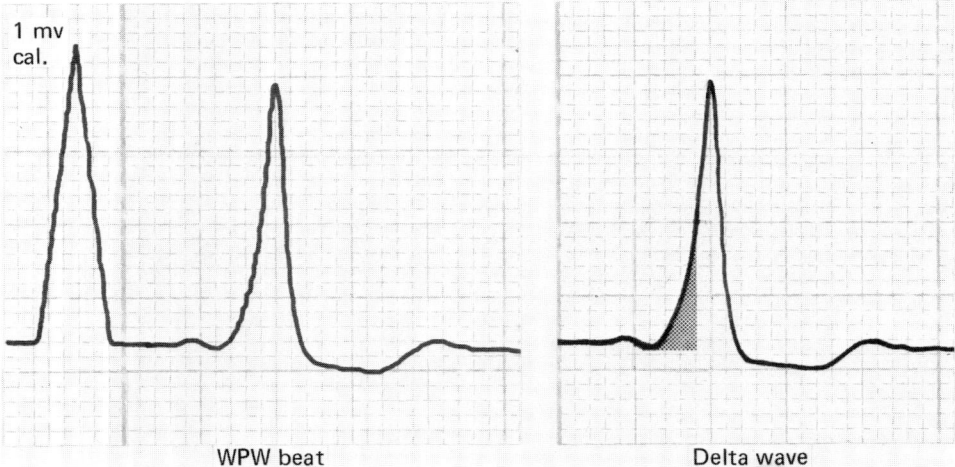

Figure 5-15.

the left ventricle (horizontal hatching) are depolarized by the impulse going normally through the AV node. This combination (actually, fusion) of early slow ventricular depolarization and normal, rapid ventricular depolarization causes the typical electrocardiographic pattern of Wolff-Parkinson-White syndrome shown in Figure 5-15.

The slurred, first part of the QRS complex which results from slow depolarization is called a *delta wave*. Frequently, the delta wave begins even before the P wave ends, so that no PR segment is present. However, the *diagnostic criteria for Wolff-Parkinson-White syndrome* are a delta wave and an abnormally short PR interval (.11 second or less) in the presence of sinus rhythm.

The size of the delta wave in a patient with Wolff-Parkinson-White syndrome depends on the amount of ventricular myocardium depolarized via the bypass tract. This, in turn, depends on the relative speed of conduction over the bypass tract and through the AV node. For example, where the bypass tract conducts much faster than the AV node, the bypassing impulse may depolarize the entire heart, and the delta wave will be very large. If, for some reason, the bypass tract conducts more slowly than the AV node, there will be no delta wave at all. In practice, changes are frequently seen in the relative speed of conduction of these two pathways, so that many patients with Wolff-Parkinson-White syndrome shift back and forth from normal to Wolff-Parkinson-White beats, and show beat-to-beat variation in the size of the delta wave. When the delta wave comes and goes in a gradual sequence, it is called the *concertina phenomenon* (Figure 5-16).

Lown-Ganong-Levine Syndrome

The Lown-Ganong-Levine syndrome is another form of preexcitation. Again the AV node is bypassed, but here the accessory pathway enters the Bundle of His (see Figure 5-17). Since the short-circuited impulse enters the Bundle of His, ventricular conduction is normal. For the same reason, when the sinoatrial impulse emerges from the AV node, it is blocked because the bypassing impulse has made the Bundle of His refractory. Therefore, the *diagnostic criteria for the Lown-*

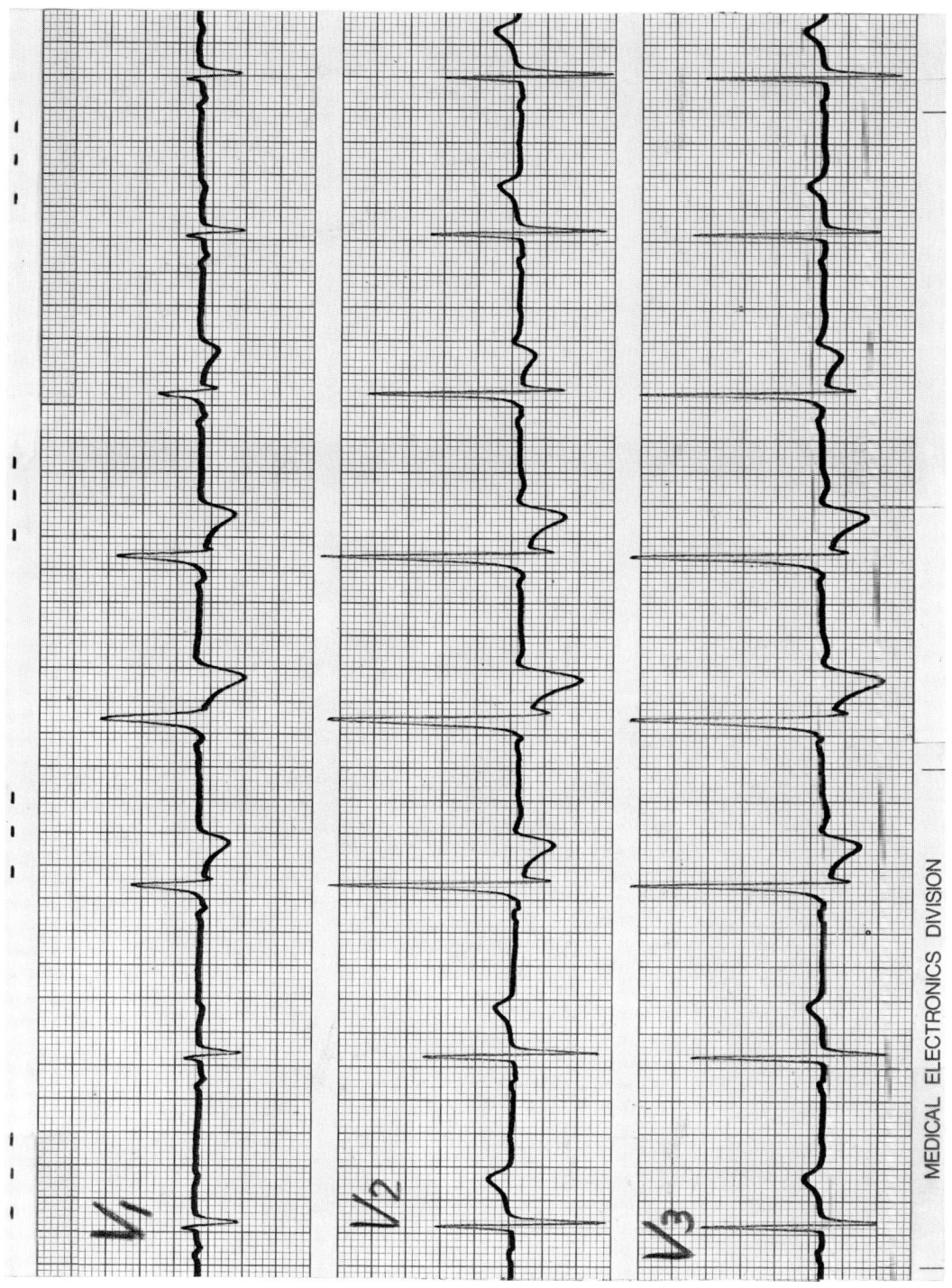

Figure 5-16.

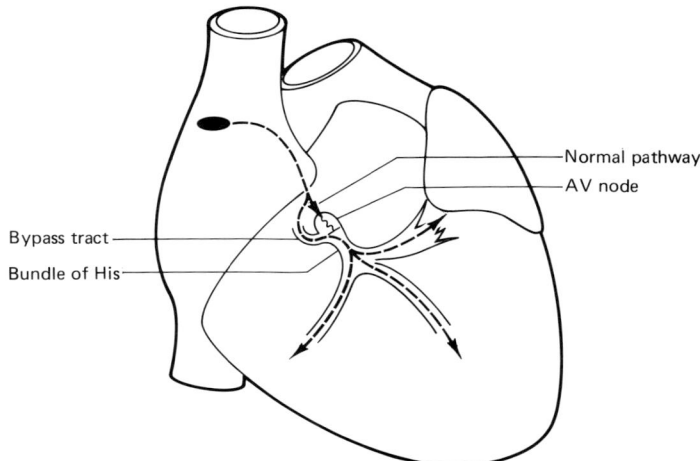

Figure 5-17. Lown-Ganong-Levine syndrome.

Ganong-Levine syndrome are an abnormally short PR interval (.11 second or less) and a QRS complex without a delta wave in the presence of sinus rhythm.

Mechanism of Arrhythmias in Preexcitation

The combination of a bypass tract and the normal conducting system creates a circuit which is capable of conducting an impulse around and around in a circus movement just like that described in the section on atrial flutter. All that is needed to start a paroxysm of tachycardia is a premature beat arising anywhere in the heart but critically timed so that it enters one limb of the circuit while the other is refractory. This situation is diagrammed in Figure 5-18, where a premature atrial impulse (1) is conducted toward the bypass tract, but blocked at (2) because the tract is still refractory from the previous normal beat. The same impulse is conducted to the AV node (3), which is not completely refractory, so it conducts the impulse to the His-Purkinje system (4) and the impulse depolarizes the ventricles. As

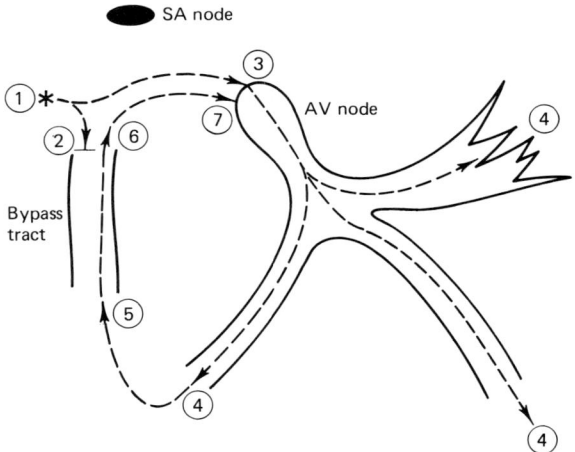

Figure 5-18. Pathway of reentrant impulse in preexcitation (Wolff-Parkinson-White).

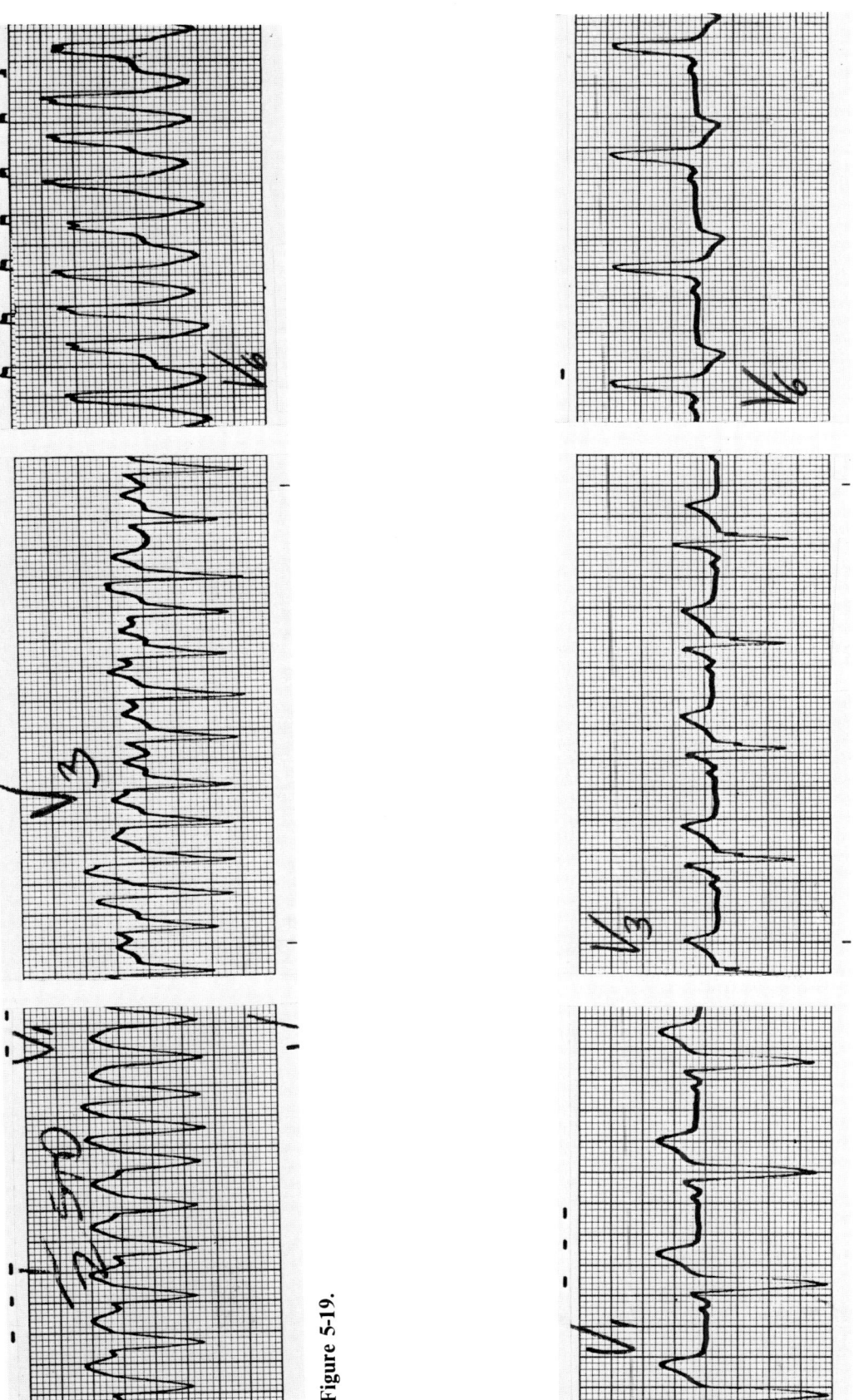

Figure 5-19.

Figure 5-20.

the ventricle adjacent to the bypass tract (5) depolarizes, the impulse enters the bypass tract, is conducted across and reenters the atrium at (6) because the time it took the impulse to travel from (1) to (5) allowed the bypass tract time to repolarize itself.

After emerging from the atrial end of the tract, the reentrant impulse spreads through the atrium, causing another P wave, and eventually reaches the AV node again (7). If the timing has been perfect, the AV node conducts the impulse into the ventricles and the circuit repeats itself. The result is a regular, paroxysmal supraventricular tachycardia. Notice that in the example shown with the impulse going retrograde through the bypass tract and antegrade through the AV node, the QRS complexes will not have a delta wave, so it will be impossible to diagnose Wolff-Parkinson-White syndrome until the tachycardia stops.

Atrial Fibrillation in Wolff-Parkinson-White Syndrome

Atrial fibrillation can be a dangerous rhythm in patients with preexcitation. Ordinarily, the AV node limits the ventricular response to 160–180 beats per minute in cases of paroxysmal atrial fibrillation. However, if the bypass tract has a shorter refractory period than the AV node, then the safety-valve effect of the AV node is lost, and 200 to 300 or more impulses may reach the ventricles each minute. Even an otherwise healthy heart cannot function properly at such a rate; so syncope, shock or even ventricular fibrillation and death may result. Furthermore, digitalis (see Chapter 6), which is usually the most effective drug for slowing the ventricular rate in atrial fibrillation, is dangerous in atrial fibrillation with Wolff-Parkinson-White syndrome because it shortens the refractory period of cardiac muscle (including the bypass tract). Therefore, the possibility of preexcitation should be considered when a patient appears with atrial fibrillation and a ventricular rate of 200 or more per minute. If it is a case of Wolff-Parkinson-White syndrome, and the atrial impulses are reaching the ventricles by way of the accessory pathway, the QRS complex will have a delta wave.

Figure 5-19 shows leads V_1, V_3 and V_6 from the electrocardiogram of a 24-year-old man who complained of rapid heart beat and near

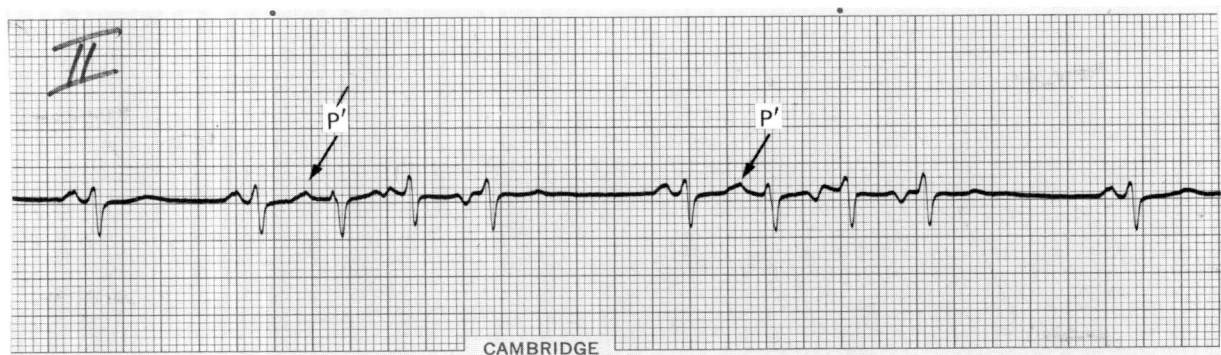

Figure 5-21.

fainting. The rapid and irregular heart rhythm should be easily diagnosable as atrial fibrillation. The unusual aspects are the extreme rapidity of the rate (RR intervals as short as .2 second, equivalent to a rate of 300 per minute) and the wide QRS complexes. These findings were suspicious of Wolff-Parkinson-White syndrome, but the definitive diagnosis could not be established until the patient was shocked into sinus rhythm. Figure 5-20 shows the same patient in sinus rhythm. The PR interval of .09 second and the prominent delta wave, best seen in lead V_3, are diagnostic of Wolff-Parkinson-White syndrome. If you think of the possibility in a patient with very rapid atrial fibrillation and carefully examine the electrocardiogram with Wolff-Parkinson-White syndrome in mind, you are not likely to miss the diagnosis.

Implications of Preexcitation for the Genesis of Cardiac Arrhythmias in Other Patients

In recent years, specialized studies of the heart have indicated that many patients with recurrent tachyarrhythmias but without electrocardiographic evidence of preexcitation have accessory pathways within the normal conduction system so that they, too, may have reentrant beats and tachycardias. Ventricular and supraventricular tachycardias may be reentrant, and the conduction pathway of the arrhythmia would look just like that diagrammed in Figure 5-18. In one of the more common types of reentrant arrhythmias, reentry occurs within the AV node itself with the impulse going down one

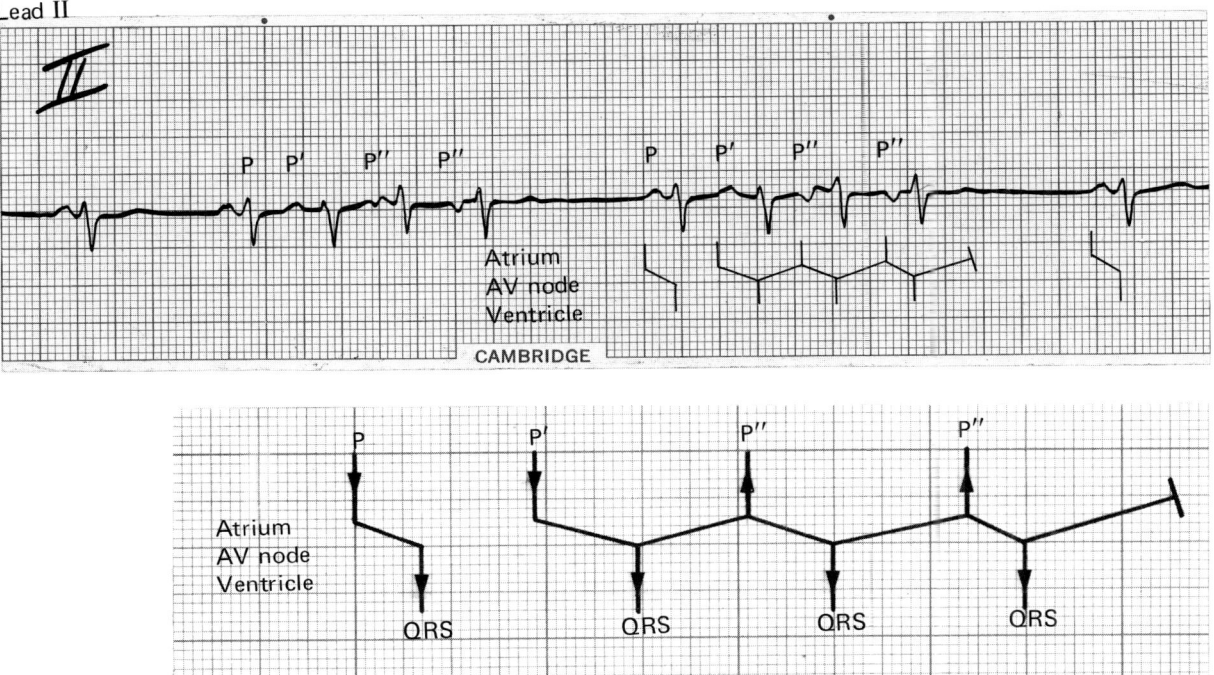

Figure 5-22.

142 / Basic Electrocardiography Handbook

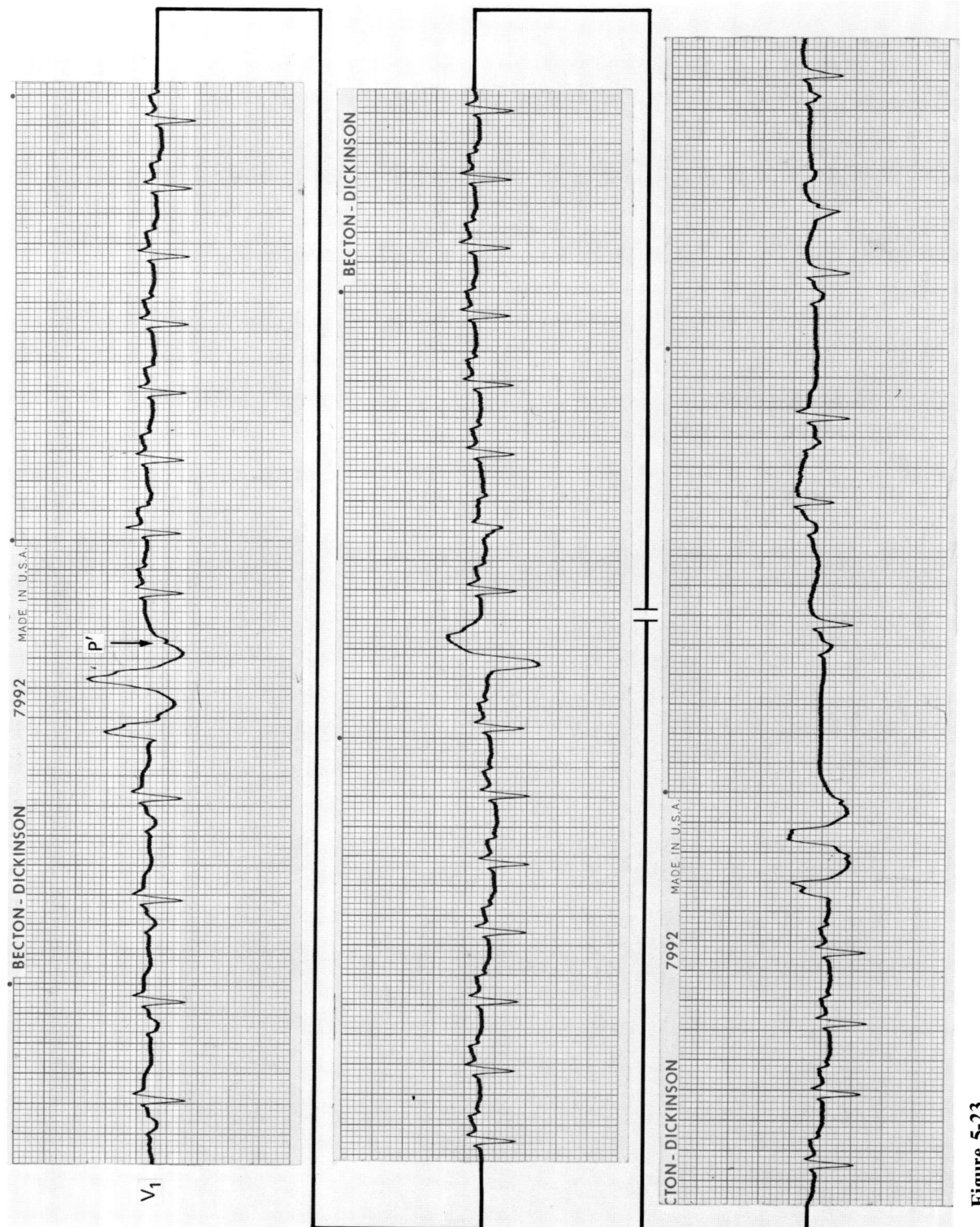

Figure 5-23.

pathway and up the other. All that is required to start such a rhythm is a properly timed premature beat.

Figure 5-21 shows two three-beat paroxysms of supraventricular tachycardia, initiated in each case by an atrial premature beat (P′) but sustained by reentry within the AV node. The diagram in Figure 5-22 shows the impulse's pathway and illustrates how a normal-looking QRS complex results when the impulse reaches the lower end of the AV node, and how a retrograde P (P″, Figure 5-22) results each time the impulse emerges from the upper end of the AV node. Figure 5-23 is a final example showing that properly timed ventricular premature beats are capable of initiating a reentrant supraventricular tachycardia. After four beats of sinus rhythm there is a salvo of ventricular premature beats. Notice the retrograde P wave (P′), which appears as a notch on the T wave of the second VPB, and begins a paroxysm of supraventricular tachycardia which continues despite single VPB's on the second strip until it is finally terminated by another salvo of VPB's in the third strip. The finding that a tachycardia can be initiated and terminated by premature beats from another part of the heart is strong evidence that the tachycardia is caused by reentry rather than enhanced automaticity.

Chapter 6
Digitalis

"Digitalis" is not a single drug, but refers to any one of a group of compounds that can be extracted from the leaves of the foxglove (*Digitalis purpurea*) and closely related plant species. Digoxin and digitoxin are two of the most commonly used digitalis preparations, but there are many others. Digitalis preparations differ in their potency, routes of administration and speed of onset of action; but once they are in the body, they all have the same effects on the heart.

Digitalis is one of the most useful agents for the treatment of many forms of heart disease, so it is widely prescribed. Unfortunately, digitalis is not an easy drug to use correctly, since the proper dose varies from person to person, and even from time to time in the same person, depending on kidney function and potassium levels, among other things. Too much digitalis (*overdigitalization, digitalis intoxication*) may cause unpleasant symptoms or dangerous or even fatal arrhythmias; so recognition of digitalis intoxication is crucial to prevent more drug from being administered, aggravating the toxic reaction. Accurate tests are now available to measure blood levels of digoxin and digitoxin, and many patients who have been overdigitalized complain of nausea, vomiting, colored or blurred vision and weakness. Still, the electrocardiogram remains one of the best ways to diagnose digitalis toxicity, particularly since toxic effects on the heart may appear before any of the other signs.

Digitalis has many effects on the heart, two of which are particularly important in the treatment of various heart diseases: (1) Digitalis makes the heart muscle contract more forcefully; therefore the drug is often given to patients with signs of heart failure to strengthen the heart's pumping action. (2) Digitalis slows conduction through the AV node; thus it can slow the ventricular rate in patients with atrial fibrillation. For example, Figure 6-1a is an electrocardiogram showing atrial fibrillation with an average ventricular response of between

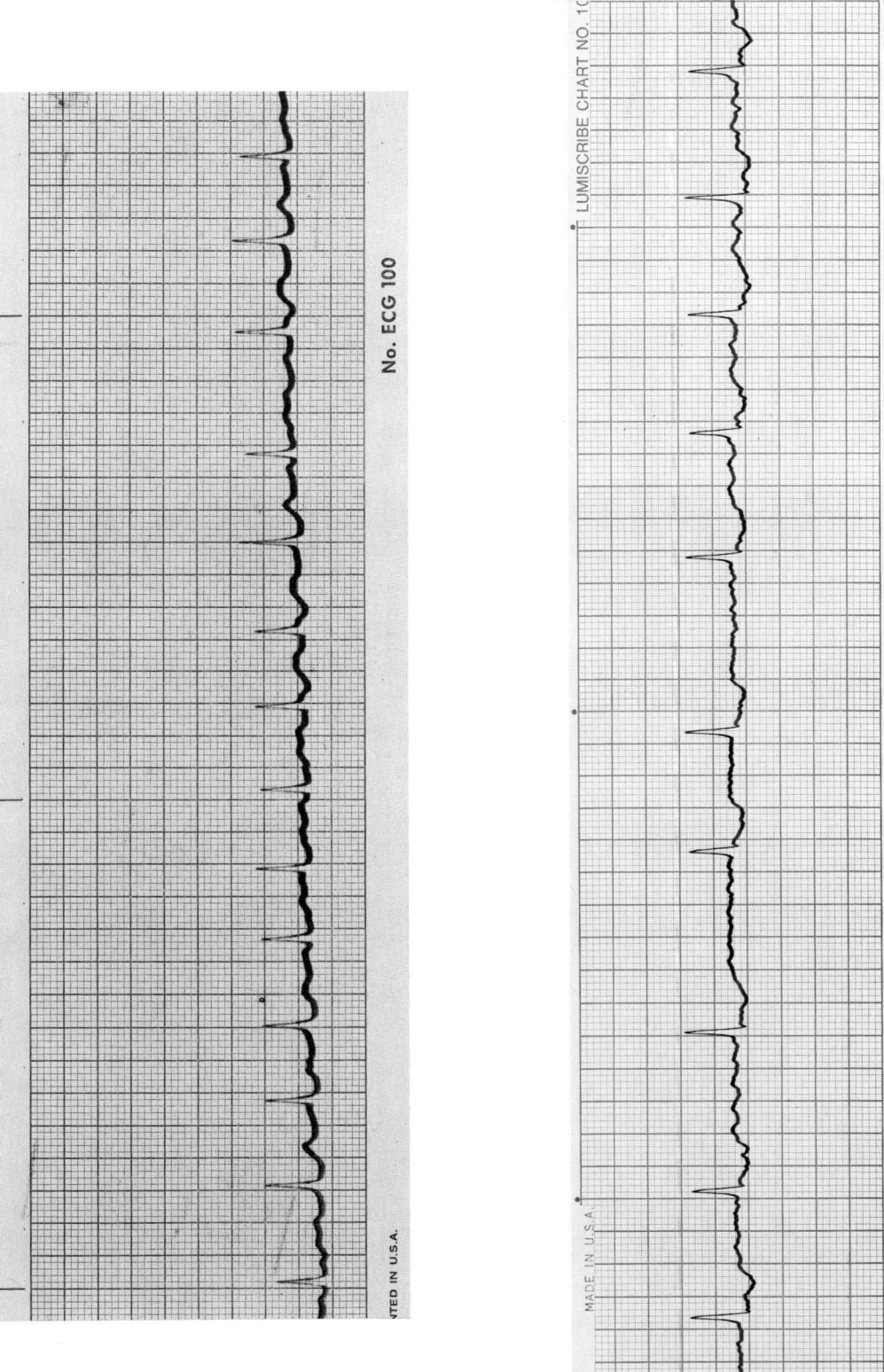

Figure 6-1b.

110 and 120 beats per minute. After the patient was treated with digitalis (Figure 6-1b), the ventricular rate slowed to between 60 and 70 beats per minute. Even though atrial fibrillation persists, the heart pumps much more efficiently at the slower rate, and the patient is much less likely to experience unpleasant palpitations. The effect of digitalis on the AV node is probably one of the reasons why the drug can often terminate paroxysmal atrial fibrillation and paroxysmal supraventricular tachycardias, restoring a regular sinus rhythm.

When Figures 6-1a and 6-1b are compared, it is evident that in addition to the slower ventricular rate in Figure 6-1b, the ST segments are more depressed and the T waves have become inverted. These changes are caused by digitalis and are often referred to as digitalis effect. Typical digitalis effects include depression of the ST segments, either as a straight line or in a sagging contour, T wave lowering or inversion and sometimes shortening of the QT interval. These changes are of no value in judging the correctness of the dosage, for they may be seen in patients who are less than fully digitalized, overdigitalized or receiving just the right amount. Similar changes may be seen on the electrocardiograms of patients with coronary artery disease, hypertensive heart disease and valvular heart disease, among other conditions; so from the electrocardiographic standpoint these are nonspecific ST and T abnormalities.

DIGITALIS TOXICITY

The abnormal rhythms seen in digitalis-intoxicated patients are the result of two effects of the drug which may occur either alone or in combination: (1) Depression of nodal tissues, including the pacemaking cells of the sinoatrial node and the conducting tissues within the AV node, occurs at therapeutic doses of digitalis but becomes much greater at toxic levels. (2) Acceleration of pacemaker cells throughout the heart occurs when toxic levels are reached.

It is often said that any cardiac arrhythmia may be caused by digitalis. While that statement is true, there are certain rhythms that are commonly caused by excessive levels of digitalis; when one or more or these occurs in a patient receiving digitalis, the possibility of digitalis intoxication should be strongly considered. The arrhythmias listed in section I of Table 6-1 are caused by depression of sinoatrial and atrioventricular nodal tissues. All of these rhythms cause slowing of the heart rate. Nurses are often taught not to administer digitalis to a patient whose heart rate is less than 60 per minute because the slow heart rate may indicate some form of digitalis toxicity.

First degree AV block is a borderline situation. It is usually not considered a sign of digitalis toxicity because most cases are not caused by digitalis. Indeed, digitalis can usually be safely prescribed for a patient who already has first degree AV block caused by underlying heart disease. However, if the PR interval becomes prolonged in a patient receiving digitalis, further administration of the drug should be done with great caution because of the possibility of causing a higher degree of AV block or other toxic rhythm. The usual procedure when digitalis has caused PR prolongation is either to stop the drug tempo-

Table 6-1. Rhythms Characteristic of Digitalis Toxicity

I. Caused by depression of nodal tissues
   1. Sinus bradycardia
   2. Sinoatrial arrest or block
   3. Type I second degree AV block
   4. Excessive slowing in atrial fibrillation
   5. Complete heart block

II. Caused by acceleration of latent pacemakers
   1. Accelerated junctional escape beats
   2. Nonparoxysmal junctional tachycardia
   3. Ventricular premature beats
      a. Bigemini
      b. Multifocal
   4. Accelerated idioventricular rhythm
   5. Ventricular tachycardia
   6. Ventricular fibrillation

III. Caused by both mechanisms
   1. Atrioventricular dissociation
   2. Paroxysmal atrial tachycardia with block

rarily or else to reduce the dose until the PR interval returns to normal At that point, if clinically indicated, the dose may again be increased but not to the level that previously caused the first degree block.

Frequently digitalis-intoxicated patients have block at the AV node (first degree, or second degree, type I) with or without junctional escape beats or an accelerated junctional rhythm. Complete or incomplete AV dissociation may ensue. If third degree AV block occurs, the escape beats are also AV junctional. Of course, these very rhythms are also typical of acute inferior infarction. Therefore, discovery of any of these rhythms on the electrocardiogram should lead to an immediate consideration of digitalis intoxication or acute inferior infarction as diagnostic possibilities.

Another finding that should strongly suggest digitalis toxicity is the appearance of ventricular arrhythmias in a patient being treated with digitalis. If a patient with atrial fibrillation has some wide QRS complexes, it is vital to determine if the wide beats represent aberrant conduction or ventricular ectopic beats or ventricular tachycardia; for ventricular ectopic beats often signify overdigitalization, while aberration is usually seen in underdigitalized patients. Application of the criteria listed in Table 3-3, Chapter 3, should lead to the correct diagnosis in almost all cases.

The pulse of a patient in atrial fibrillation is irregular, corresponding to the irregular heart action. If the patient is treated with digitalis, and the pulse becomes regular, this change may indicate something good or something bad; only the electrocardiogram can tell which. "Something good" is that regular sinus rhythm has returned. "Something bad" is that complete heart block or atrioventricular dissociation with accelerated junctional escape rhythm, nonparoxysmal junctional tachycardia, accelerated idioventricular rhythm or ventricular tachycardia has appeared because of digitalis toxicity. Therefore, always obtain an electrocardiogram when the pulse becomes regular in a patient with atrial fibrillation.

QUIZ

Review Electrocardiograms

Each of these electrocardiograms was recorded from a patient receiving digitalis. Analzye the rhythm and decide, for each case, if the patient is (a) probably underdigitalized, (b) receiving the correct dose of digitalis, (c) probably overdigitalized (digitalis-intoxicated).

Answers

Case 1. This should have been easy—the rhythm is atrial fibrillation with a ventricular response averaging over 130 per minute and no ventricular ectopic beats. The answer is (a); the patient is probably underdigitalized and should receive more digitalis until the ventricular rate slows.

Case 2. This patient is in sinus rhythm, 80 per minute. The PR interval is .28 second (first degree AV block). By itself, first degree AV block does not mean digitalis intoxication, but it should make you suspicious. In this case, multifocal ventricular premature beats are also present; so the correct answer is (c), probably overdigitalized. Notice the marked ST segment depressions caused by digitalis.

Case 3. It should be obvious that this patient with atrial fibrillation has had too much of a good thing (answer c). The ventricular response has been slowed excessively; the longest RR interval is almost 3 seconds. This patient may well have had dizzy spells or syncope.

Case 4. This rhythm strip shows a regular atrial rhythm and a slower, irregular ventricular rhythm, suggesting that second degree AV block is present. More detailed analysis indicates an atrial rate of 65 per minute with changing PR intervals. Going from left to right, the PR intervals are .32, .34, .36 and .40 second, and then a P wave is not conducted to the ventricles. This is Type I second degree AV block. The next QRS complex occurs almost simultaneously with the next P wave, which just begins to show itself before the upstroke of the R wave. This beat is a junctional escape beat. Another Wenckebach sequence follows, where the PR intervals are .30, .40 and .44 second, and then the next P is not conducted. Once again the pause is terminated by a junctional escape beat. Type I second degree AV block with or without junctional escape beats should always raise suspicion of digitalis intoxication, particularly if the patient does not have an acute inferior myocardial infarction. In this case, the diagnosis of digitalis toxicity (answer c) was confirmed by a high serum digoxin level.

Case 5. This electrocardiogram may look frightening, but it shouldn't be. When you see narrow and wide QRS complexes on the same

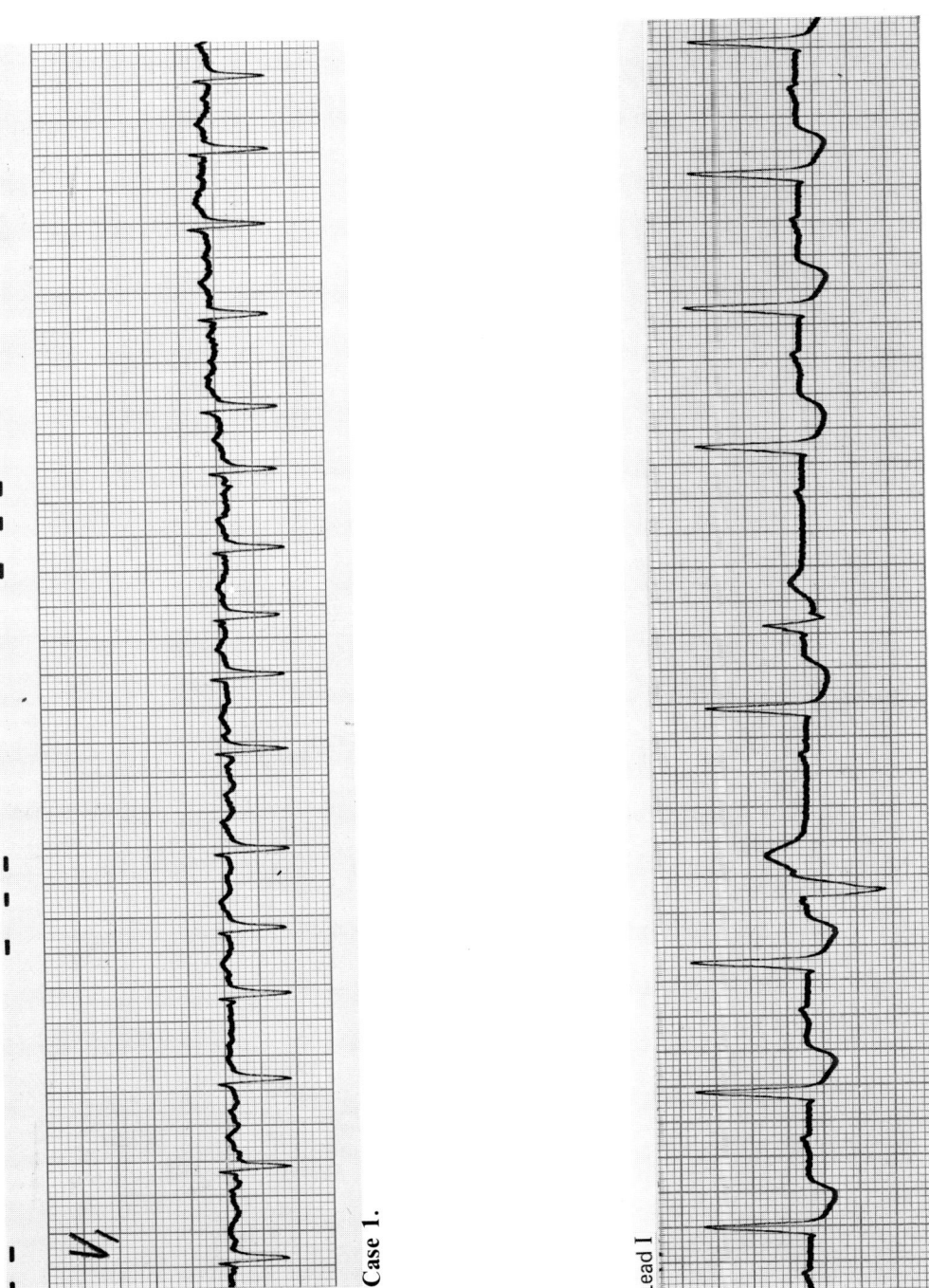

Case 1.

Case 2.

150 / Basic Electrocardiography Handbook

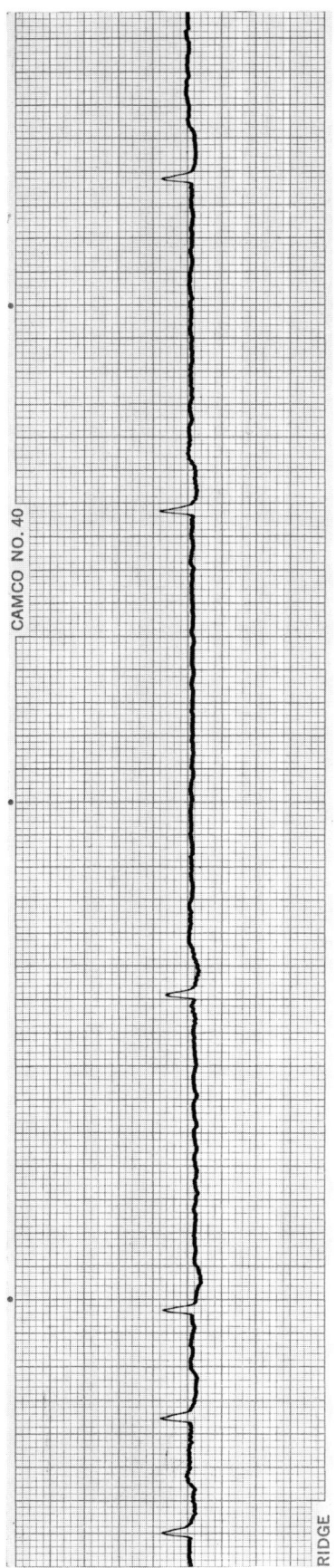

Case 3.

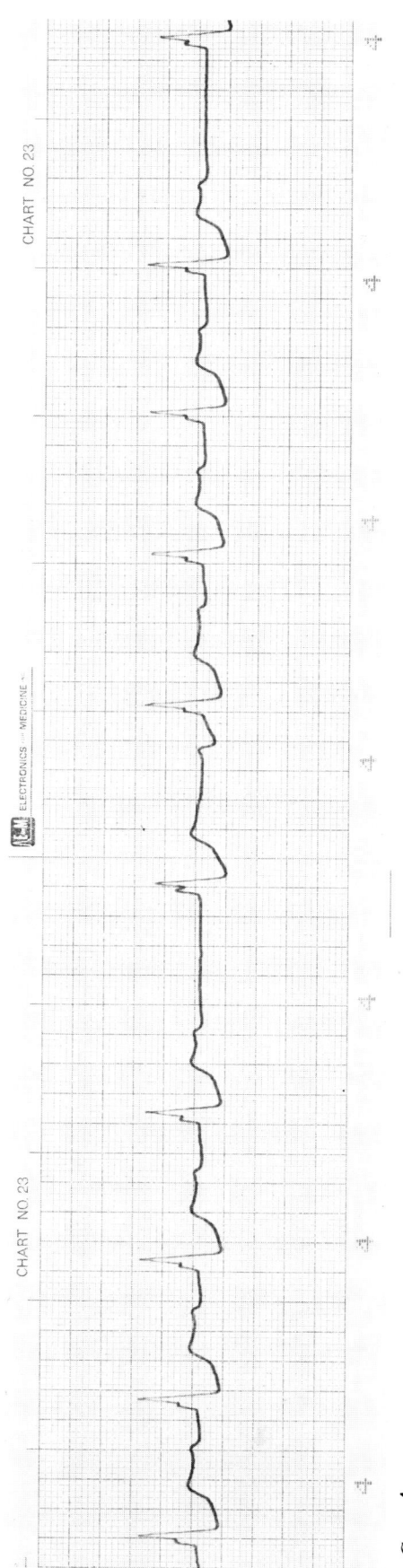

Case 4.

electrocardiogram, it is usually best to begin by analyzing the narrow complexes to determine the basic rhythm. This can be done in leads II, L, the V_1 rhythm strip at the bottom and the first half of V_2, V_3 and V_6. There we see rapid but irregular QRS complexes at an average rate of 130 per minute. There are no discrete P or flutter waves, so this must atrial fibrillation. Now there are two possibilities to consider for the sequences of wide QRS complexes—are they aberrant, or are they runs of ventricular tachycardia? Apply the criteria of Table 3-3, Chapter 3. We have already determined that the ventricular response is rapid. Does the first wide QRS complex end a short RR interval after a long one every time? Yes, it does. Are the runs of wide complexes regular or irregular? Irregular. How about the rate of the wide complexes? It's practically the same as the rate of atrial fibrillation. Finally, the configuration of the wide beats in V_1—they have the QS pattern of a left bundle branch block. Since it is neither RSR' nor QR, it doesn't help us. In summary, there are four criteria favoring aberration and none favoring ventricular ectopy, so we may conclude that this is a case of atrial fibrillation with rapid ventricular response and aberrant conduction. This patient needs more digitalis (answer a).

Incidentally, if you happened to notice the wide Q waves in III and F, and ST segment elevations plus T wave inversions in II, III, F, V_5 and V_6, and, therefore, diagnosed an acute inferolateral myocardial infarction, you may go to the head of the class.

Case 6. If you correctly diagnosed the rhythm, you knew what to do about the digitalis. There are rapid and regular P waves at a rate of 160 per minute, and regular, narrow (hence, supraventricular) QRS complexes at 135 per minute. Two regular rhythms at different rates with changing PR intervals can occur only if the atria and ventricles are beating independently. In other words, atrioventricular dissociation is present, and the correct answer is (c). Contrast this tracing with case 4, where the combination of a regular atrial rhythm and slower *irregular* ventricular rhythm indicated that AV conduction was taking place, but abnormally because of the toxic effect of digitalis on the AV node.

Case 7. This is a case of atrial fibrillation where the rhythm became regular at 72 beats per minute after treatment with digitalis. This electrocardiogram was taken to see whether the patient had been cured of her atrial fibrillation or overdosed with digitalis. You can see from the wavy baseline without distinct P waves that atrial fibrillation persists. Except for the salvo of ventricular premature beats at the end of lead II (another finding suggesting digitalis toxicity), the QRS complexes have a rapid upstroke and downstroke of the R wave, indicating a supraventricular origin even though the QRS duration is .13 second. Since the atria are fibrillating, the beats must be originating in the AV junctional tissues. This is AV dissociation, not complete heart block, because the junctional pacemaker is going faster than 60/minute. If you also diagnosed nonparoxysmal junctional tachycardia, so much the better. But whether you diagnosed this as AV dissociation, nonparoxysmal junctional tachycardia or both, you

152 / Basic Electrocardiography Handbook

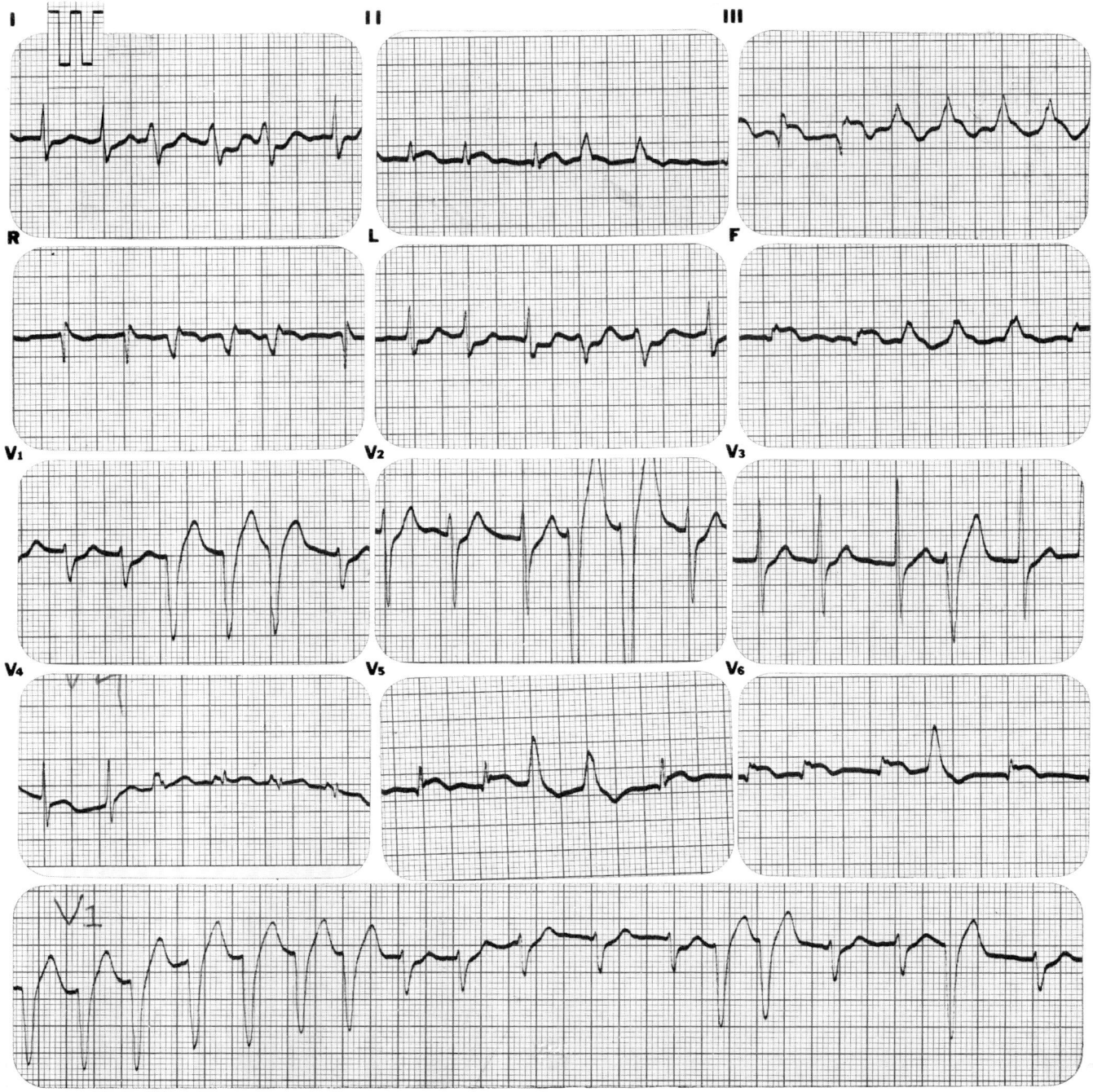

Case 5.

must have recognized this as another example of overdigitalization (answer c).

Case 8. Case 8 shows what may happen when even small doses of digitalis are given to hypokalemic patients. Strip *A*, a sample of lead V_1 before any digitalis was given, shows sinus rhythm at 88 per minute. A few hours after a single, relatively small dose of digoxin—

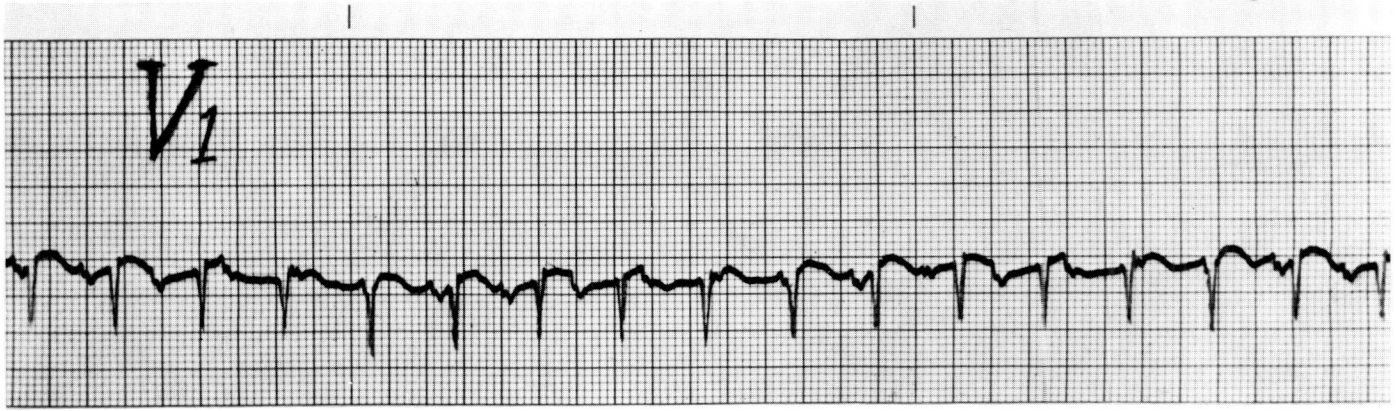

Case 6.

only half the usual digitalizing dose—the rhythm abruptly changed to an atrial tachycardia with regular P waves at 135 per minute. The change in P configuration confirms that the atria are no longer under the control of the sinoatrial node. Throughout most of strips *A* and *B* there are two P waves for every QRS, indicating that 2:1 block is present. Paroxysmal atrial tachycardia with block is an uncommon arrhythmia, but about two-thirds of the cases are caused by digitalis toxicity (answer c). The simultaneous appearance of ventricular premature beats is further evidence of digitalis toxicity. Fortunately,

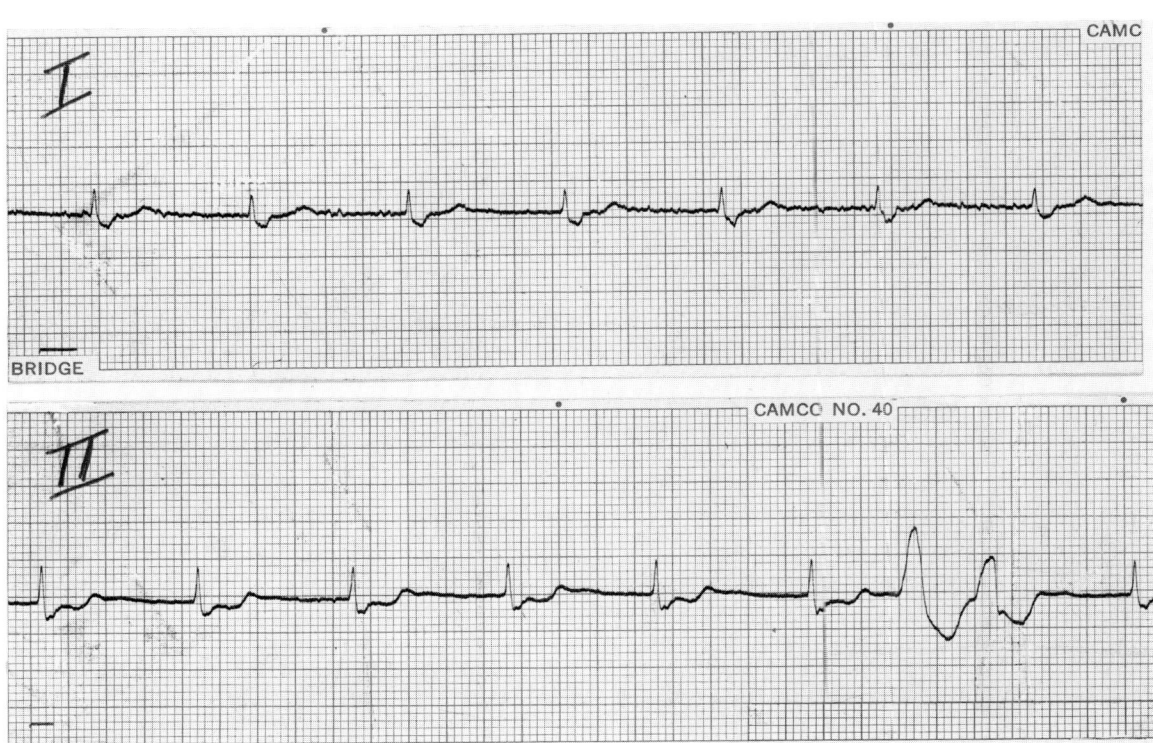

Case 7.

154 / **Basic Electrocardiography Handbook**

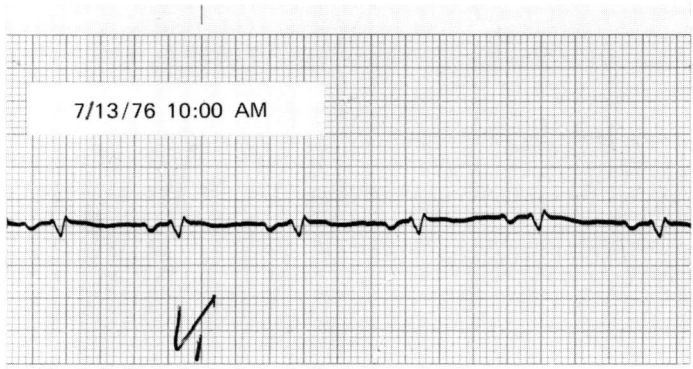

7/13 PM 0.5 mg digoxin intravenously

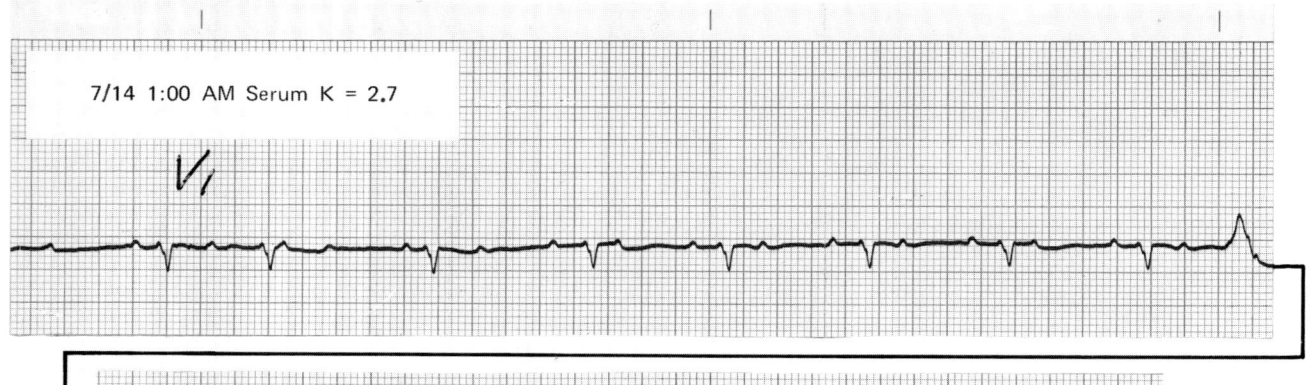

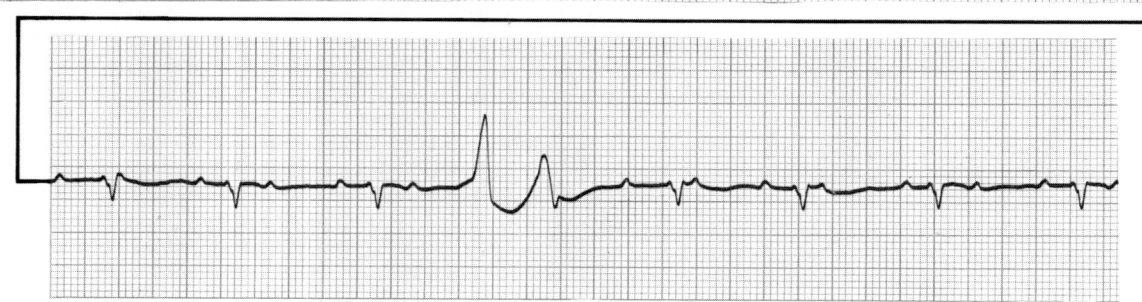

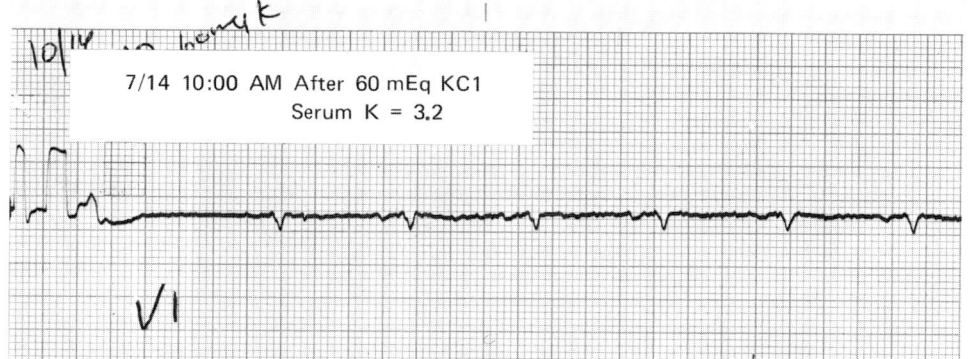

Case 8.

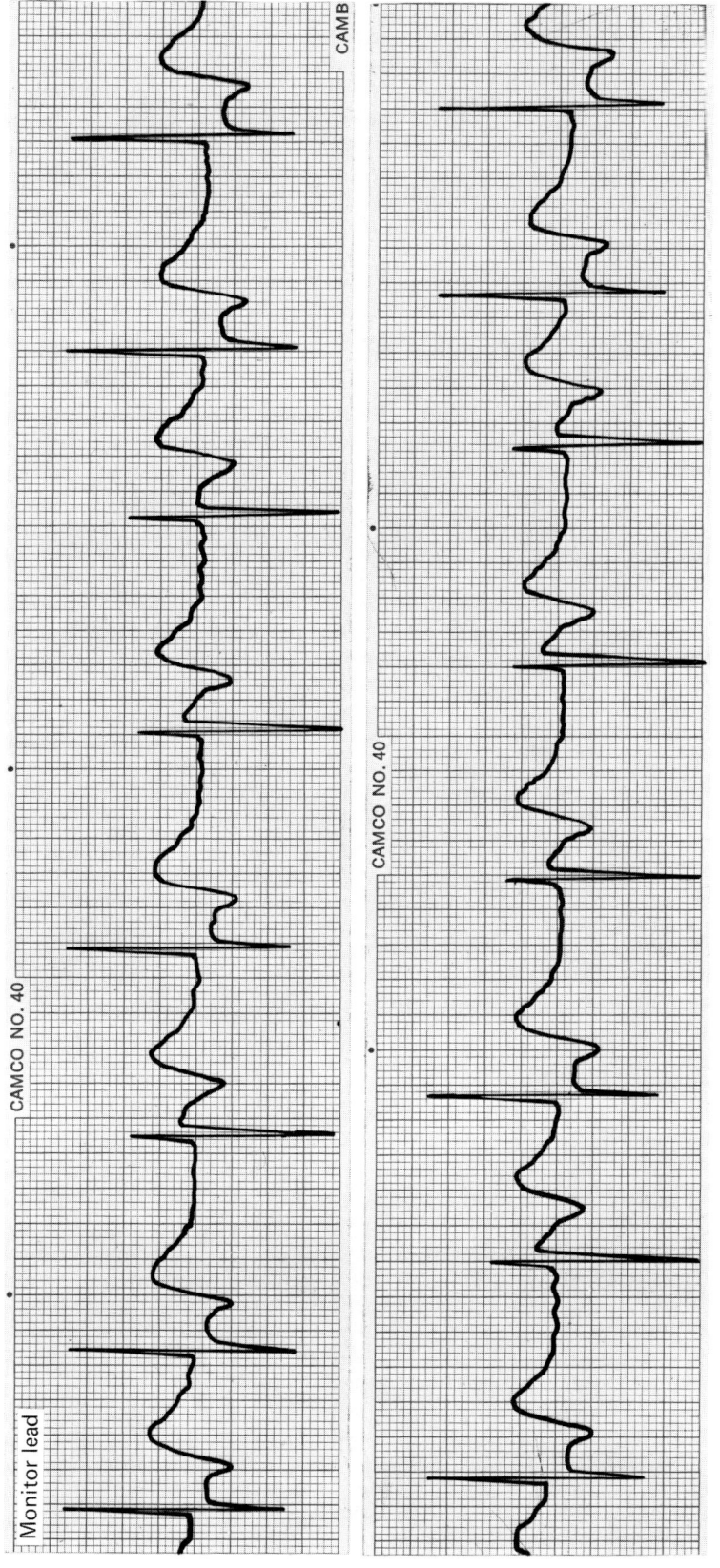

Case 9.

even though it was one o'clock in the morning, the physicians on the case realized that a low serum potassium had made this patient unusually sensitive to digitalis, so that only a small dose of digoxin resulted in a toxic rhythm. The patient was then given potassium intravenously, and of course no more digoxin. By 10 A.M. (strip C) the patient was back in regular sinus rhythm; notice that the P waves have changed back to their normal pattern as shown before in strip A.

Case 9. This is a subtle but common example of digitoxicity (answer c) that is all too often overlooked. From the undulating baseline, and the overall irregularity, it should be easy enough to diagnose this as a case of atrial fibrillation. However, the ventricular rhythm is not completely irregular. Also, there are two different QRS patterns—one with R larger than S, the second with S larger than R. The RR interval as measured between beats with the first type of QRS complex varies, as expected in atrial fibrillation. However, the RR interval between two of the second type of beat is always 1.24 seconds.

It is not possible to have a regular ventricular rhythm in uncomplicated atrial fibrillation. It can only happen with complete heart block (Figure 3-27, Chapter 3) or AV dissociation (Case 7). But what about a partly regular rhythm, as in this case? If the RR interval between the regular beats is longer than the longest RR interval between irregular beats, then the regular beats must be escape beats. Since the QRS complexes of the regular beats are less than .12 second in duration, they must be supraventricular. Since they can't be atrial—remember, the atria are fibrillating—they must be AV junctional. Slight aberration is not unusual with AV junctional beats (Figure 3-9, Chapter 3). Since their rate is 48 per minute, they are not accelerated junctional escape beats. Nevertheless, there must be considerable AV block if these junctional beats have the opportunity to escape; so this is an example of excessively slow rate in atrial fibrillation plus AV junctional escape beats, and that should add up to a diagnosis of too much digitalis.

In this particular case, the patient had advanced kidney disease, and was being treated with digoxin, which can only leave the body via the kidneys. Even though the dose given was small, a toxic level accumulated. It might have been wiser to treat this patient with digitoxin, which is mostly eliminated through the liver, and, therefore, less likely to intoxicate a patient with kidney disease.

Chapter 7
Pacemakers

More and more patients are being treated with artificial pacemakers. A pacemaker rhythm looks different from anything else on an electrocardiogram, and the electrocardiogram often gives the first signs when a pacemaker is not working properly. This chapter will review the principles of artificial pacing, a few commonly used types of pacemakers and their effects on the electrocardiogram and finally some electrocardiographic signs of pacemaker malfunction.

PRINCIPLES AND USES

Most of the time, pacemakers are used to treat patients with symptomatic bradycardias or, particularly in some patients with acute myocardial infarction, patients who are at high risk of developing dangerous bradycardias such as complete heart block. Occasionally pacemakers are used to try to control tachycardias that fail to respond to drug therapy.

Although there are many types of pacemakers, all work on the general principles diagrammed in Figure 7-1. The pacemaker consists of a source of electric power, usually batteries, connected to the heart by an insulated wire, the *pacing catheter*. Each time the pacemaker gives off an electric signal, actually a small shock, the signal is conducted down the catheter to the heart. Let us say the catheter is inside the right ventricle, as it would be in the majority of patients being paced nowadays. The pacemaker impulse stimulates the right ventricular myocardium next to the catheter; then the impulse spreads into the His-Purkinje system and is conducted through the right and left ventricles, causing the heart to contract. If the pacemaker fires 70 times a minute, the heart will beat 70 times a minute.

Those familiar with electrical devices know that there must be a path for the current to return to the source, to complete the elec-

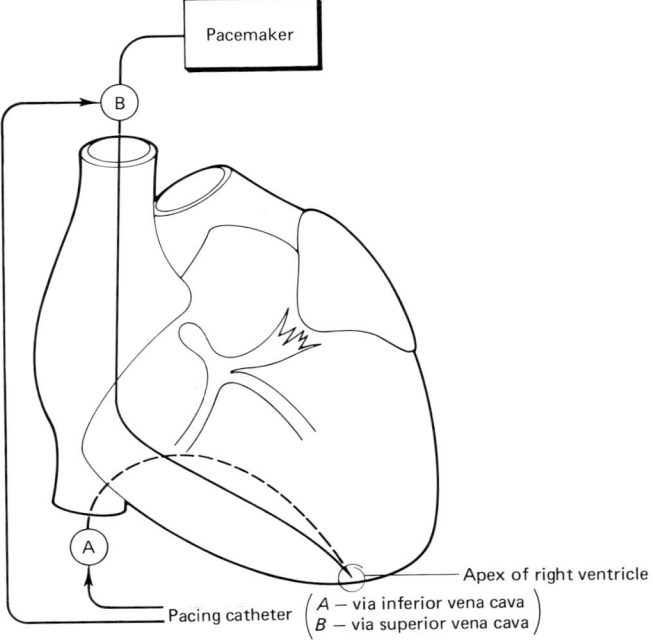

Figure 7-1.

trical circuit. The circuit may be completed in one of two ways, depending on the type of catheter used. If there is only one wire in the catheter, it is called a *unipolar catheter* (Figure 7-2A). Current flows down the catheter to the heart, then back through the body tissues of the chest in order to reach the other electrical terminal, a metal plate on the pacemaker itself or a second wire attached to the skin. A *bipolar catheter* contains two wires, one ending at the tip of the catheter, the other one-half inch or so behind it. In this type the current flows out the tip of the catheter and returns to the pacemaker by way of the other wire in the catheter (Figure 7-2B). There are advantages and disadvantages to each type of catheter; but with proper technique, each type works well, and both types of catheters are widely used.

A permanent pacemaker is implanted in the body, just under the skin so that it can be removed and replaced easily when the batteries run down. Only the pacemaker is replaced. Barring a wire

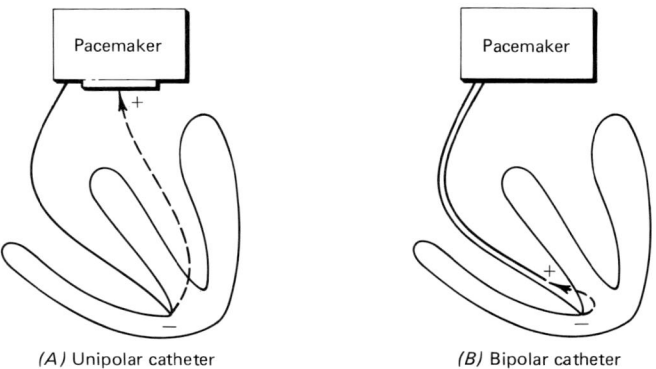

Figure 7-2.

break (*fracture*) or other malfunction, the same catheter is used for the life of the patient. A *temporary* (or *external*) *pacemaker* remains outside the body, with the catheter coming out through the skin to be connected to the temporary pacemaker. When the pacemaker is outside the patient, it is a simple matter to change the rate of pacing or the strength of the pacing stimulus according to the patient's needs. Temporary pacing is rarely used for more than a few days or weeks. The main indications for temporary pacing are (1) to stabilize a patient's rhythm before a permanent pacemaker is implanted; (2) to treat a condition that requires pacing which is not expected to last long, for example, a bradycardia complicating acute myocardial infarction; (3) as a trial to see whether a patient improves by being paced before proceeding with a permanent pacemaker implantation.

Figure 7-3 is a rhythm strip showing a typical pacemaker electrocardiogram. Each QRS complex is preceded by a sharp deflection called a *pacemaker spike*, which represents the pacing stimulus. The size of the spike varies, depending on which lead is recorded. Its size will increase as the stimulus is increased. Also, pacemakers with unipolar catheters register larger spikes than those with bipolar catheters. In fact, the large spikes recorded from unipolar pacemakers often return so slowly to the baseline that it may be hard to determine if a QRS complex is really present. This situation is illustrated by a malfunctioning unipolar pacemaker in Figure 7-4. The rhythm strip includes five pacemaker spikes (numbered). Spikes 1, 3, 4 and 5 fail to stimulate the heart, yet each of these spikes is followed by a slow, downward wave that is much larger than the spontaneous QRS complexes. This *overshoot artefact* is not part of the pacemaker spike, but is caused by the electrocardiograph machine in response to the sudden, large stylus deflection caused by the pacemaker spike. The overshoot artefact can be mistaken for a QRS complex if you are not careful. However, notice the difference between these overshoot artefacts and the true QRS complex following the second spike, which appears as a notch in the overshoot artefact and is followed by a prominent T wave. Occasionally a catastrophe occurs when an observer notes large pacemaker spikes with overshoot artefacts on a monitor and mistakenly assumes everything is satisfactory when, in fact, the patient is in asystole or ventricular fibrillation.

In many cases, the condition requiring pacemaker therapy comes and goes, so that for at least part of the time the patient's own heart beats faster than the pacemaker's rate. If the pacemaker is a *fixed-rate pacemaker* (one that continues to fire at its preset rate no matter what the patient's heart is doing), the result is *competition*, a situation where two pacemakers (one natural, one artificial) compete for control of the heart. Competition may cause several undesirable side effects, the most drastic of which is ventricular fibrillation, which may result if a pacemaker stimulus reaches the ventricle during the vulnerable period of the previous normal beat. For this reason most pacemakers in current use are *noncompetitive* (*demand*) *pacemakers*. These pacemakers are equipped with sensing circuits

160 / Basic Electrocardiography Handbook

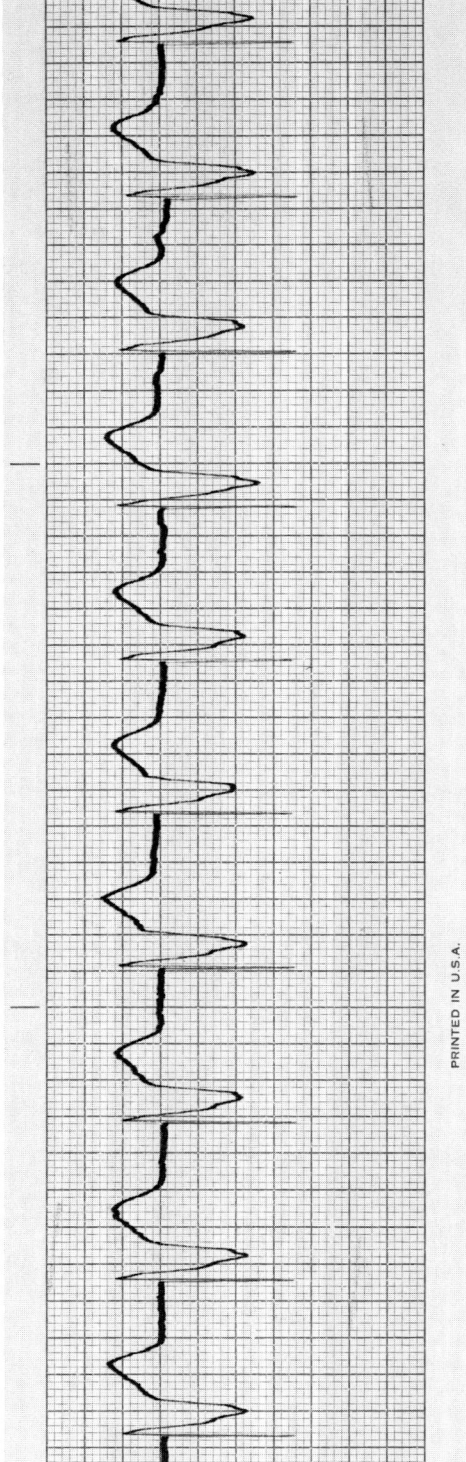

Figure 7-3.

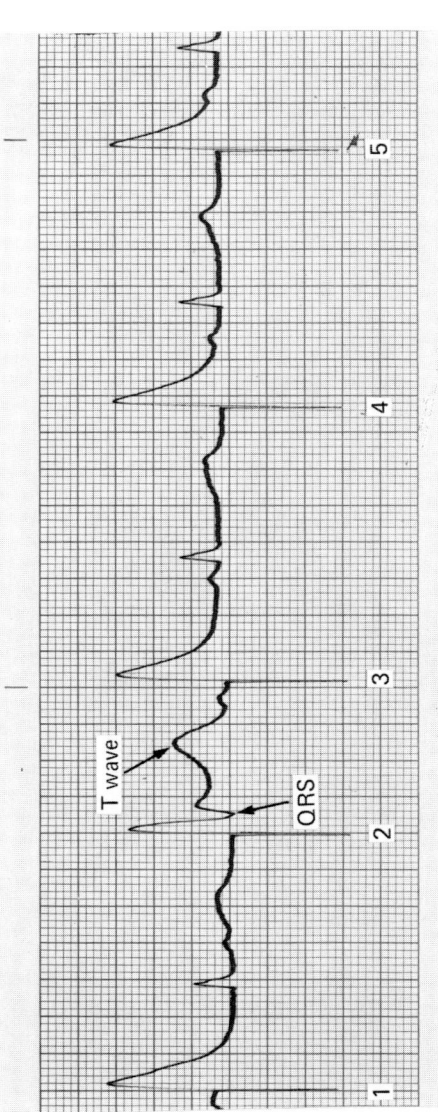

Figure 7-4.

that enable the pacemaker to recognize a normal heart beat and stop the pacemaker from firing until the patient's own heart becomes slower than the pacemaker's rate.

Figure 7-5 is a rhythm strip recorded from a patient with a noncompetitive pacemaker whose escape rate is 60 per minute. The first two beats are normal sinus beats at 62 per minute. This rate is just fast enough to *inhibit* (turn off) the pacing circuit, so there are no spikes until after the third P wave. The reason that the pacemaker began to fire is that the sinus rate slowed to 56 per minute. Since the pacemaker did not detect another QRS complex within one second (the interval between beats at a rate of 60 per minute) of the second QRS on the strip, the pacemaker's firing circuit was not inhibited; so pacing stimuli began to appear. This type of noncompetitive pacer is called a *ventricular inhibited pacemaker* because spontaneous ventricular complexes inhibit the pacemaker. This is the most common type of pacemaker in use today. If you understand its principles, you can understand any kind of pacemaker just by knowing whether the pacer is fixed-rate or noncompetitive and to which chamber(s) of the heart the pacing catheter(s) go.

RECOGNIZING PACEMAKER MALFUNCTION

A fixed-rate pacemaker has only one function, pacing, while a noncompetitive pacer has two, sensing and pacing. A properly functioning pacemaker should do what it is supposed to do all of the time, not just most of the time. For example, failure to pace for even a few beats may be the first sign of a problem that, if uncorrected, might lead to total failure of the pacemaker.

Figure 7-6 shows a fixed-rate pacemaker set at 60 per minute, competing with a sinus rhythm at 78 per minute. The third and seventh pacemaker spikes are not followed by QRS complexes Is this pacing failure? No, because both spikes come before the T wave of the previous QRS complex, that is, during the ventricle's absolute refractory period. Therefore, we *diagnose pacing failure* only when spikes falling outside the ventricular refractory period fail to cause a QRS complex. Incidentally, did you recognize the eighth QRS complex as a fusion beat? Fusion beats are common in patients with artificial pacemakers, particularly when the spontaneous heart rate is close to that of the pacemaker. The third QRS in Figure 7-5 is also a fusion beat.

Figure 7-7 shows a properly functioning noncompetitive pacer set at 60 per minute. Each paced QRS is followed by a ventricular premature beat. From each ventricular premature beat it is about five large boxes (one second) to the next paced beat, showing that the pacemaker has been reset by the premature beat. Contrast this with Figure 7-6 where the patient's own beats fail to reset the pacemaker.

Figure 7-8 was recorded from a patient whose ventricular inhibited pacemaker was set at 70 per minute. There should be little difficulty in recognizing this as a case of pacing failure, since the large,

162 / **Basic Electrocardiography Handbook**

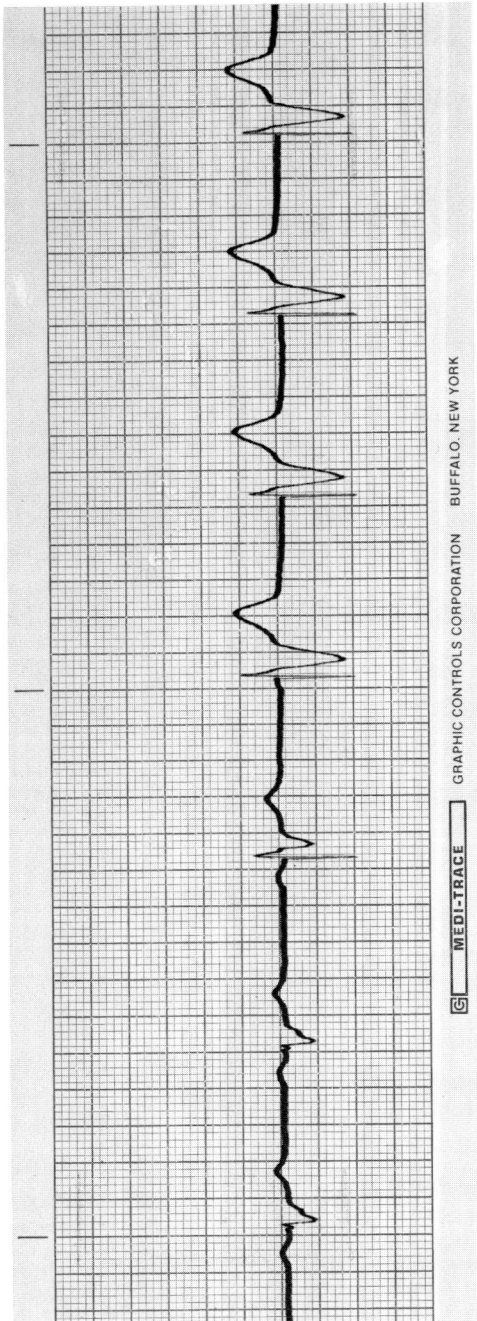

Figure 7-5.

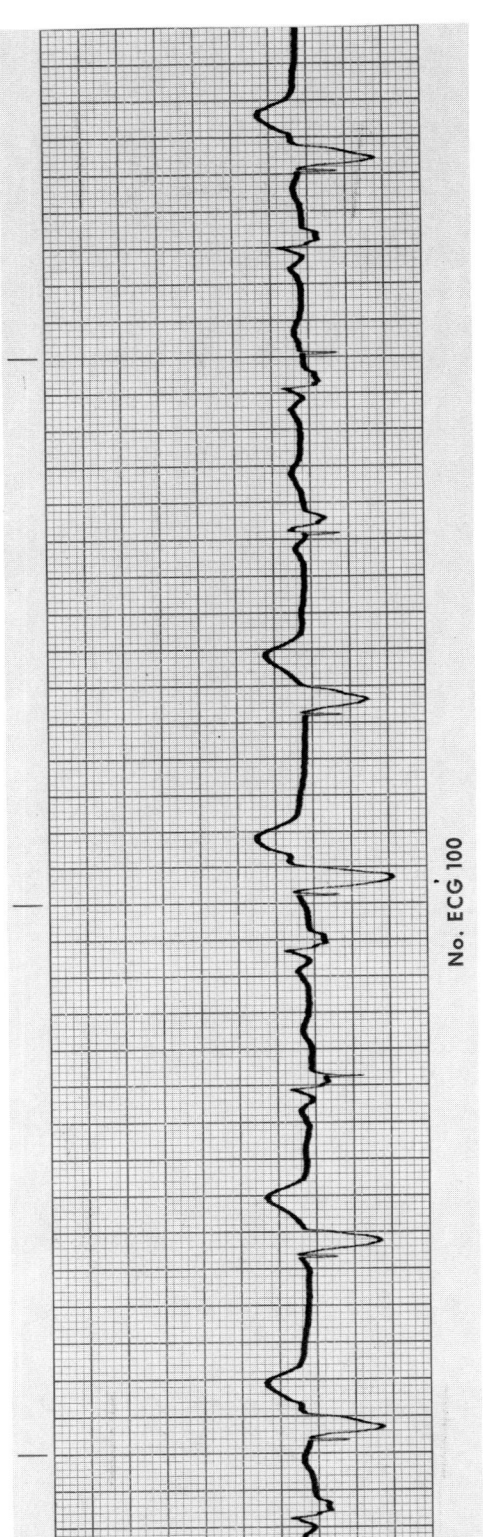

Figure 7-6.

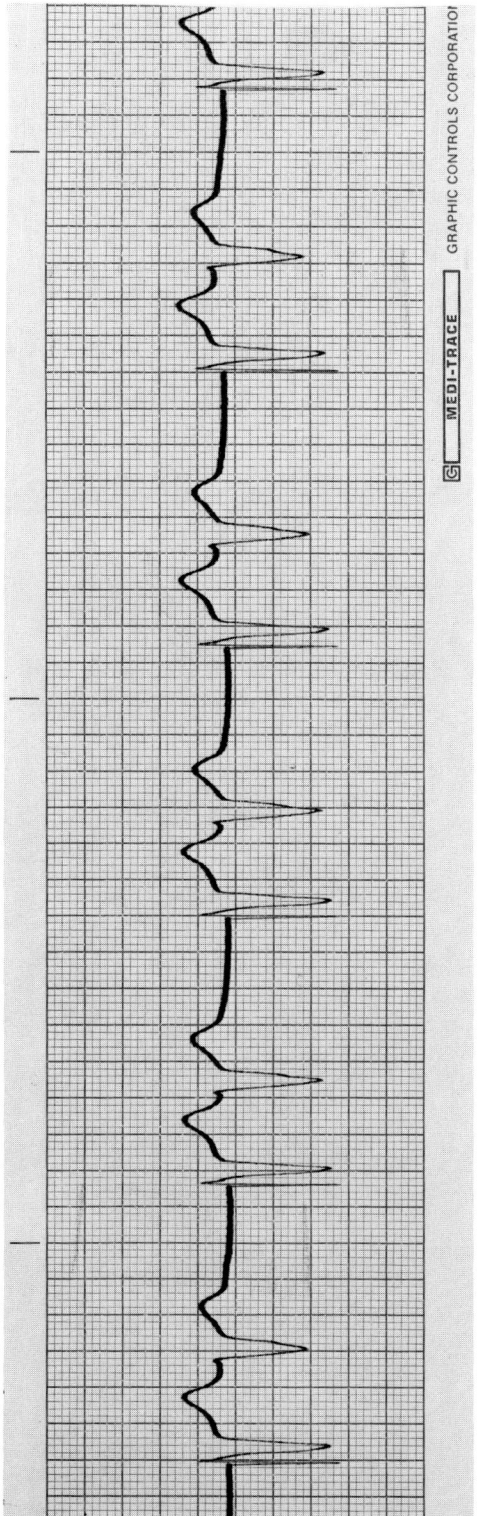

Figure 7-7.

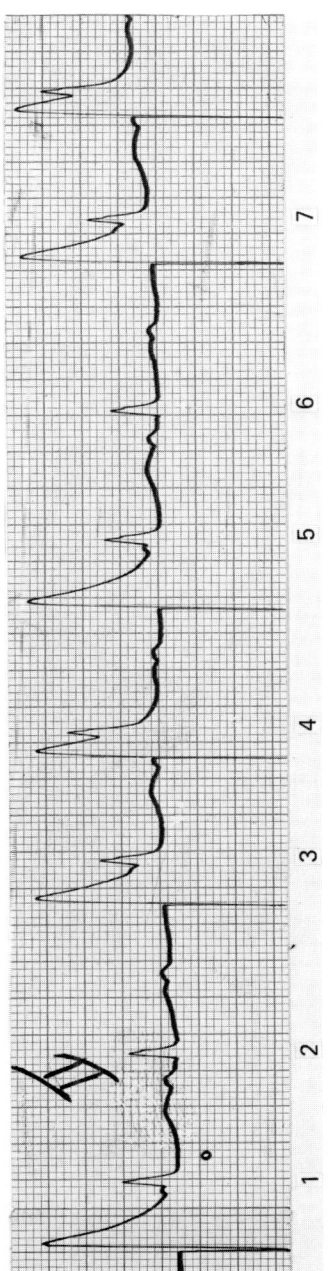

Figure 7-8.

Table 7-1. Diagnosis of Pacemaker Malfunction

Malfunction	Diagnostic criteria
Pacing failure	Some or all pacemaker stimuli falling outside the ventricular refractory period fail to elicit a QRS complex.
Sensing failure	Some or all spontaneous QRS complexes falling outside the pacemaker's refractory period fail to inhibit pacemaker firing. (For ventricular triggered pacemakers, some or all spontaneous QRS complexes falling outside the pacemaker's refractory period fail to trigger the pacemaker.)

unipolar pacing spikes are followed only by the fall-off artefact and not by a QRS complex and T wave. The problem is, is sensing normal or is sensing failure also present?

QRS complexes 1, 2, 5 and 6 are sensed by the pacemaker because no pacemaker spike is seen for at least .85 second after those beats (.85 second is the RR interval for a rate of 70 per minute). Complexes 3, 4 and 7 are not sensed. However, notice that complexes 3, 4 and 7 are closer to the pacemaker spike than 1, 2, 5 and 6. All noncompetitive pacemakers are designed with a refractory period for their sensing circuits, so they will not be affected by the pacemaker spike. The duration of the refractory period varies from model to model, but usually is between .2 and .4 second. Therefore, beats 3, 4 and 7 were not sensed because they fell during the pacemaker's refractory period; so they do not indicate any abnormality of sensing function. To *diagnose sensing failure*, we must find QRS complexes outside the pacemaker's refractory period that fail to inhibit the pacemaker.

Table 7-2. Some Causes of Pacemaker Malfunction

Problems with the catheter
    Malposition (improper placement in heart)
    Dislodgment (movement from original, correct position)
    Perforation of the heart
    Heavy fibrosis around catheter tip
    Fracture of wire
    Break in insulation
    Small endocardial QRS complexes
    Improper sealing of catheter—pacemaker connection

Problems with the pacemaker
    Battery depletion
    Leakage of body fluids into pacemaker
    Component failure (including faulty manufacture)
    Detection of noncardiac electric currents from
        chest muscles, home appliances such as microwave
        ovens, electric tooth brushes, electric razors, etc.
    Short circuit between pacemaker terminals

Criteria for diagnosis of pacing and sensing failure are summarized in Table 7-1.

There are, unfortunately, many different problems that may affect the pacing catheter or the pacemaker itself and lead to sensing failure, pacing failure or both. Table 7-2 lists some of these potential problems. Some of these diagnoses are easy to make; others may be difficult, requiring elaborate electronic equipment. The important thing is to recognize that a malfunction exists and promptly notify the persons responsible for care of the pacemaker.

BATTERY DEPLETION IN PERMANENT PACEMAKERS

After a period of time, all pacemakers will fail because their power source (batteries, nuclear generator, etc.) will run down and fail to deliver enough current to stimulate the heart. When this happens, the patient usually resumes whatever heart rhythm was present before the pacemaker was implanted. If that rhythm happened to be complete heart block or some other severe bradycardia, syncope or sudden death might occur. Therefore, every effort must be made to replace pacemakers before they fail, but not before they begin to lose their power. For this reason, most permanent pacemakers are designed to change their rate as battery power begins to fall. A rate change of five beats per minute or more from the basic rate—normally determined about four months after implantation to allow for slight rate changes caused by "settling in"—means a significant drop in battery power and indicates that the pacemaker unit should be replaced. Figure 7-9 shows lead II strips taken one month (*upper*) 13 months (*middle*) and 15 months (*lower*) after pacemaker implantation. The first two show fixed-rate pacing at 70 per minute, while the third shows that the pacing rate has slowed to 58 per minute. Notice, too, that the pacemaker spike has become smaller—another, although less dependable, indication of loss of power. Do not be misled because the pacemaker is still pacing—with this kind of a rate change, the pacer will fail completely within a few days or weeks.

PACEMAKER FOLLOW-UP

With the proliferation of pacemaker manufacturers and models, the task of following up pacemaker patients has become increasingly complex. While gross malfunctions and major rate changes are detectable by standard electrocardiograms, the detection of slight but important fluctuations in pacemaker rate, output and stimulus wave form requires much more sophisticated equipment. Optimal permanent pacemaker follow-up requires regular visits to and/or regular telephone checks by a properly equipped facility supervised by physician(s) knowledgeable in pacemaker technology. The performance of periodic electrocardiograms on pacemaker patients is not as good a follow-up, but it is a lot better than no follow-up at all or the automatic replacement of the pacemaker after an arbitrary period of time.

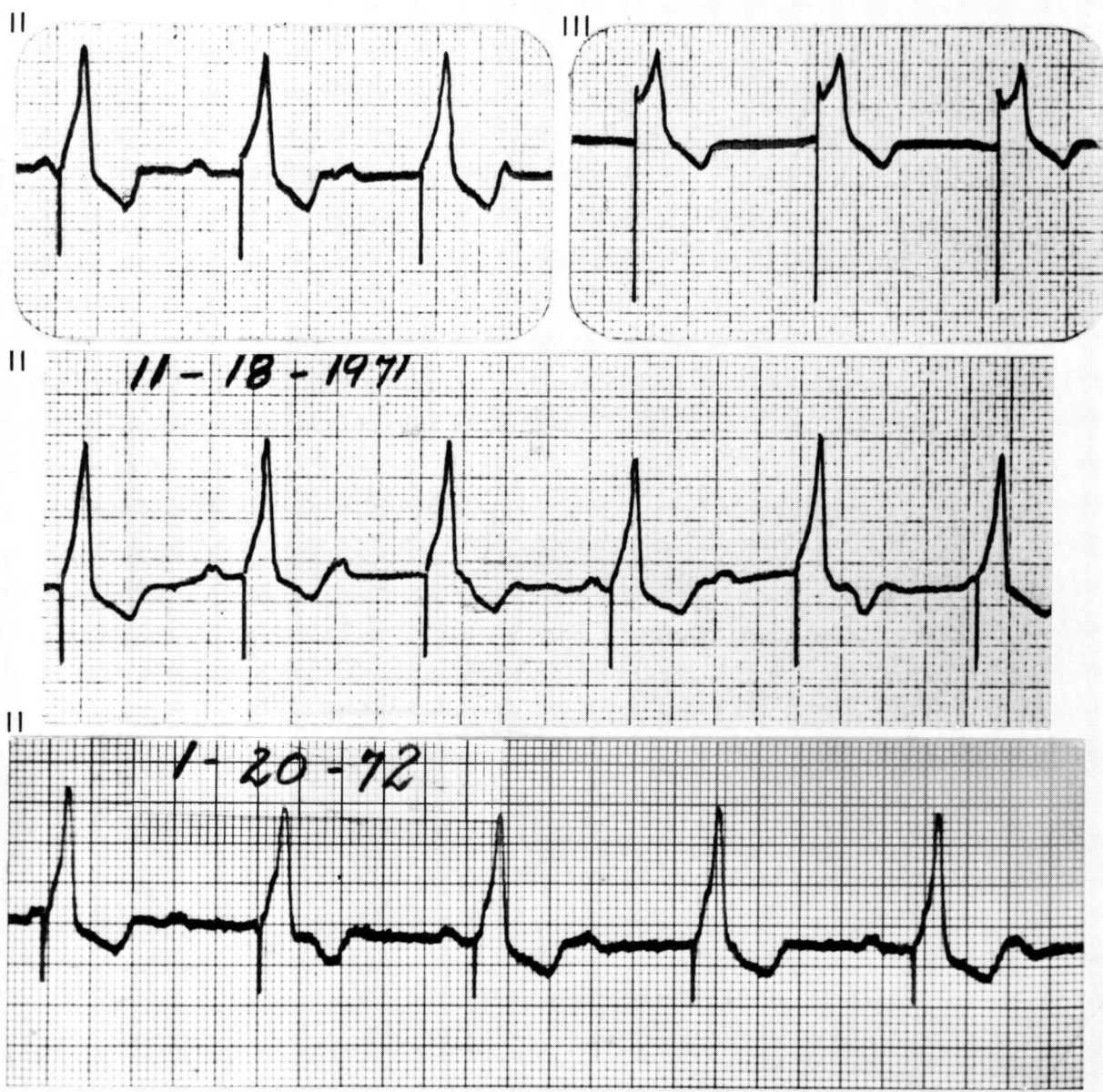

Figure 7-9.

CORRECTION OF MALFUNCTIONS

When a permanent pacemaker malfunction is detected, there is little the noncardiologist can do besides call for help, except possibly administer drugs to try and stabilize the patient's own heart rate. With a temporary pacemaker, however, the pacemaker controls and connections to the catheter are outside the body. This means that in case of emergency, anyone familiar with the pacemaker controls can make a possibly life-saving adjustment.

There are two types of temporary pacemaker malfunctions (Table 7-3) where do-it-yourself repairs should be tried while the respon-

Table 7-3. First Aid for Malfunctioning Temporary Pacemakers

Condition	Treatment
Pacing failure, spikes present	Turn up pacer output
Pacing failure, spikes absent	Tighten all connections Look for short circuit Make sure pacemaker has been turned on Turn up pacer output Try another pacemaker with fresh battery

In any case, notify the pacemaker specialist who is following the patient.

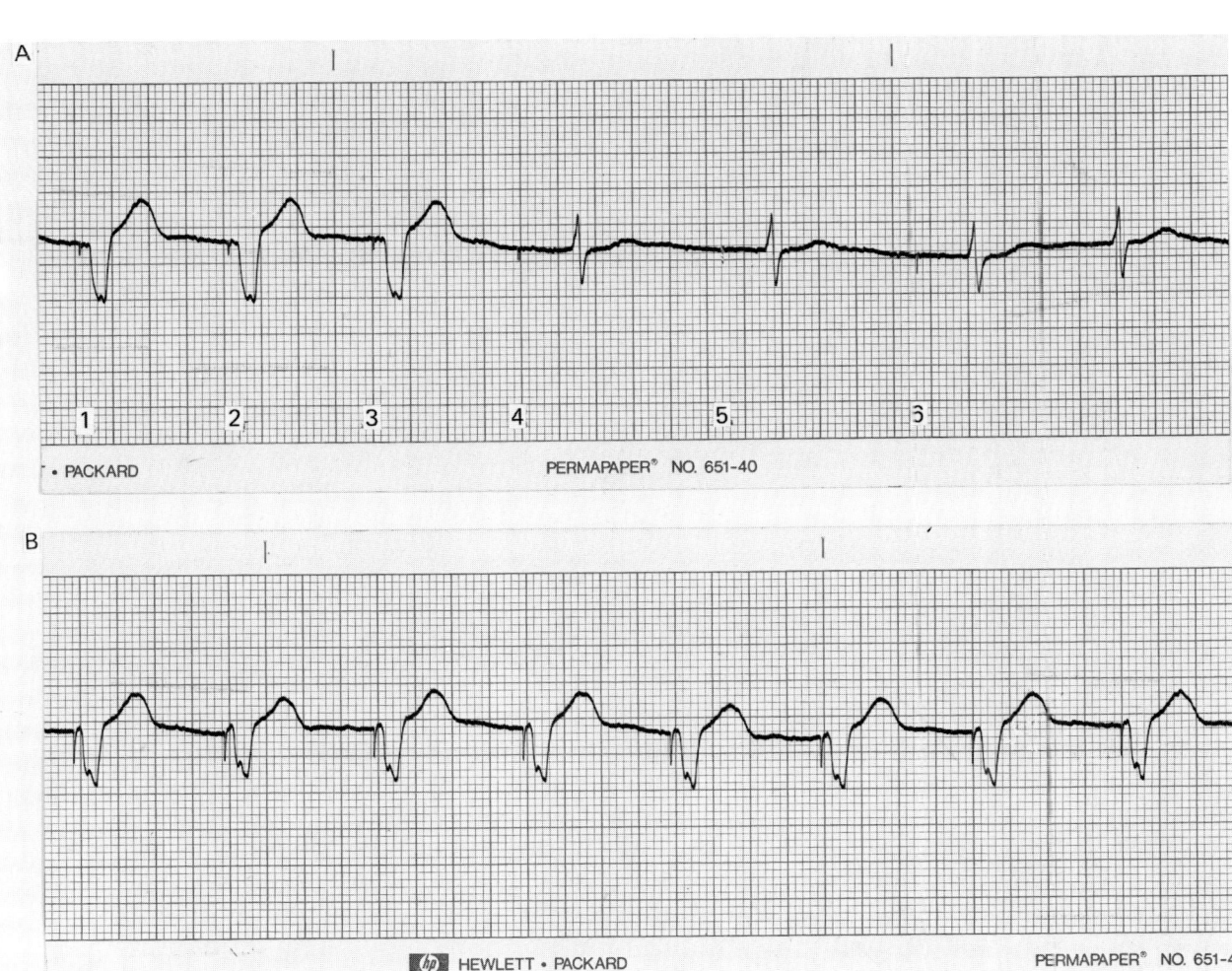

Figure 7-10.

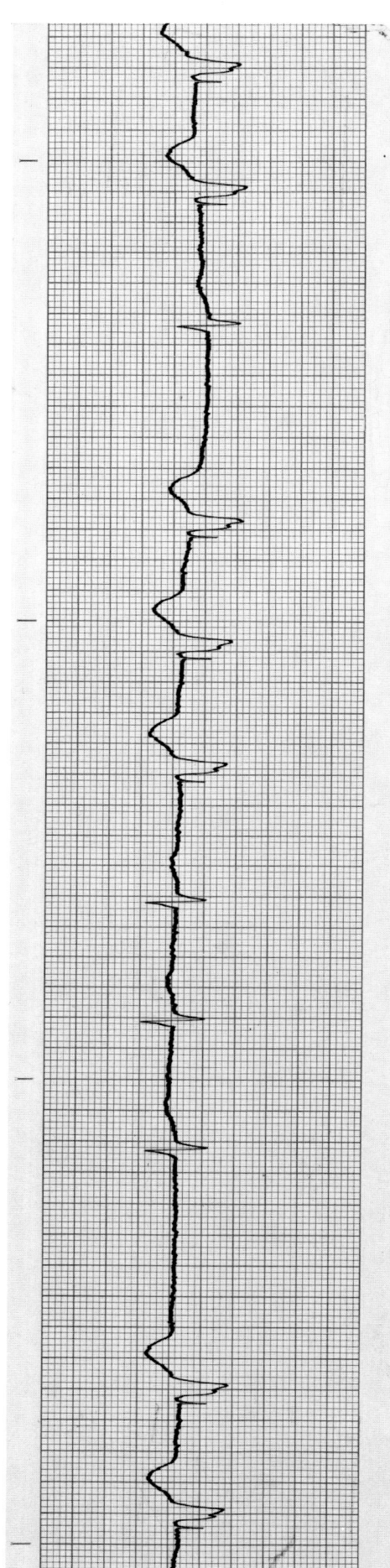

Figure 7-11.

sible physician is being contacted, the first of which is pacing failure with pacemaker spikes visible on the EKG. There are two common causes for this finding: (1) an inflammatory reaction in the heart around the tip of the catheter may increase the ventricular *stimulation threshold* (the lowest amount of current that will cause the ventricles to contract) so that the pacemaker output is no longer sufficient to stimulate the heart (this complication is also known as *pacemaker exit block*); (2) the catheter may become dislodged so that it is no longer in contact with the right ventricular endocardium. In this situation, try turning up the current that the pacemaker delivers; this will restore pacing if exit block is the problem, but it will do nothing either good or bad if the catheter is dislodged, since in that case, the current is no longer being effectively delivered to the ventricle.

Figure 7-10A is a rhythm strip showing pacemaker exit block recorded from a patient with a temporary pacemaker. The first three pacemaker spikes result in QRS complexes, but 4, 5 and 6 do not. Notice, however, the delayed appearance of spikes 5 and 6, indicating that the pacemaker did sense the patient's spontaneous beats. Strip *B* was recorded after the pacemaker's electrical output was increased. Normal pacemaker function was restored. Notice, too, the increased size of the spikes, reflecting the increased output.

There are many possible causes of pacing failure without pacemaker spikes. When the condition is intermittent, as is shown in Figure 7-11, there are two readily corrected causes that should be immediately looked for. One is a break in the circuit, caused by a loose connection between the pacemaker catheter and the pacemaker. Sometimes an extension cable or adaptor is placed between the catheter and the pacemaker; it increases the possibility of a loose connection. Therefore, begin by making sure that all connections are tight. Another easily corrected cause of this type of malfunction is a short circuit caused by a wire touching both pacemaker terminals. It is particularly likely to occur with unipolar, temporary pacemakers when the wire to the skin is not insulated with tape and touches both terminals of the pacemaker at once or the uninsulated part of the pacing catheter. Elimination of the short circuit will immediately restore pacing.

If the pacing failure is not intermittent, and there are no spikes seen at all, a loose connection or a short circuit may still be responsible. But there is another possibility—someone may have turned the pacemaker off, either intentionally or accidentally; so be certain that the pacemaker is switched on.

In some cases of exit block, the pacer spikes are so small that you may not see them and may conclude they are absent altogether. Therefore, if you can't find a loose connection, there is no short circuit and the pacemaker is on, try turning up the output. Pacing failure without spikes may also be caused by a loose connection or broken wire within the pacemaker itself (*component failure*). If so, you can restore pacing by attaching another pacemaker with a fresh battery to the pacing catheter. This maneuver will also correct the situation if the battery of the first pacemaker had run down, causing a drop in electrical output.

Unfortunately, sensing failure in a temporary pacemaker is not so easily corrected, since in most cases the problem is with the catheter or its placement in the heart. However, two adjustments can be made to solve the problem temporarily, particularly if there are complications resulting from the competing rhythms: (1) Turn the pacemaker off; this will eliminate competition, but if bradycardia or asystole occurs, you must remember to turn the pacemaker on again. (2) Increase the pacemaker rate to 5–10 beats per minute faster than the spontaneous rhythm. Since the fastest pacemaker controls the heart, this maneuver usually replaces the competitive rhythm with a more rapid pacemaker rhythm. However, except in extraordinary cases neither of these adjustments should be performed without consulting the pacemaker specialist following the patient.

Appendix

This appendix replaces the usual glossary. The key words and terms listed below are defined in the text on the pages indicated.

aberrant conduction, 50
accelerated rhythm, 47
antegrade, 51
anterior, 5
aortic valve, 1
arrhythmia, 8
atrioventricular block, 26
atrioventricular junction, 25
atrioventricular dissociation, 28
atrioventricular node, 25
atrium (plural, atria), 1
automaticity, 47
axis, 11

bifascicular block, 40
bigeminal rhythm, 54
bipolar, 158
bradycardia. 44
Bundle of His, 26

capture beat, 78
cardiac output, 48
circus movement, 47
compensatory pause, 56
competition, 159
component failure, 169
concertina phenomenon, 136
contraction (of the heart), 1
coronary blood vessels, 3

deflection, 2
delta wave, 136
demand pacemaker, 159

depolarization, 3
diastole, 1

ectopic rhythm, 45
effusion, 121
electrical alternans, 121
electrocardiogram, 2
electrocardiograph, 2
electrode, 6
electrode fracture, 159
embolus, 122
endocardium, 2
endothelium, 3
epicardium, 3
escape beat, 30

fascicle, 26
fixed rate pacemaker, 159
fusion beat, 82

horizontal heart, 7
hypertrophy, 10

idioventricular, 32
impulse, 25
indeterminate axis, 12
infarction, 92
inhibit, 161
interval, 2
intraventricular block, 32
ischemia, 94

J point, 4

latent, 30
left bundle branch, 26
lesion, 32
Lown-Ganong-Levine syndrome, 136

mitral valve, 1
monitoring, 9
multifocal, 50
myocardial infarction, 92
myocarditis, 27
myocardium, 3

overshoot artefact, 159

P wave, 3
pacemaker exit block, 169
pacemaker spike, 159
pacing catheter, 157
pacing failure, 164
paroxysmal, 44
pericarditis, 119
pericardium, 3
pleuritic (pain), 119
precordial, 8
preexcitation, 131
premature beat, 45
pulmonary valve, 1
pump failure, 97
Purkinje cells, 26

QRS complex, 3, 4

reentry, 47
refractory, 48

repolarization, 3
retrograde, 51
right bundle branch, 26

salvo, 47
segment, 2
sensing failure, 164
slurred, 34
sinoatrial node, 25
standardization, 10, 14
stimulation threshold, 169
stylus, 2
subendocardial myocardial infarction, 94
supraventricular, 30
syncope, 84
systole, 1

T wave, 3, 4
tachycardia, 44, 47
threshold, 169
transmural myocardial infarction, 93
tricuspid valve, 1
trifascicular block, 40

U wave, 4
unifocal, 50
unipolar, 158

ventricle, 1
ventricular inhibited pacemaker, 161
vertical heart, 7
vulnerable period, 87

Wenckebach phenomenon, 27
Wolff-Parkinson-White syndrome, 134

Index

AV junctional. *See* junctional
aberrant conduction, 50, 55, 59, 69–75, 148–151
accelerated idioventricular rhythm, 47, 82–84, 147
accelerated junctional escape rhythm, 47, 75–80, 147
anatomy of the heart, 1–3, 25, 26
angina pectoris, 95
aortic valve, 1
artefacts, 13–24, 159
    caused by imprecise lead placement, 17–18
    caused by incorrect standardization, 14
    caused by lead reversal, 15–17
    caused by loose electrodes, 20–23
    caused by muscle tremor, 23–24
    caused by pacemaker, 159
    caused by respiration, 18, 84
    caused by 60 cycle interference, 18–20
    caused by smeared electrode paste, 18
atrial fibrillation, 65–75, 87, 147–152, 156
    in preexcitation, 140–141
atrial flutter, 63–65
atrial premature beats, 48–51
atrial tachycardia, 61–63
    with block, 63, 152–156
atrioventricular block, 26–32
    caused by digitalis, 144–148
    first degree, 26–27, 42–43
    in myocardial infarction, 109–115
    second degree, 27–30
    third degree, 30–32, 69
atrioventricular dissociation, 28, 69, 80, 86, 109, 147, 151–152, 156

atrioventricular junction, 25, 30
atrioventricular node, 25, 27, 141–143
    effect of digitalis, 144–148
    in myocardial infarction, 99, 109
    in preexcitation, 131–141
atropine, 117–118
automaticity, 47
axis deviation, 11–13

bifascicular block, 40–43
    in myocardial infarction, 109–115
bigeminal rhythm, 54
bradycardia, 44
    caused by digitalis, 146–147
    in myocardial infarction, 117–118
bundle branch block, 33–38
    in myocardial infarction, 98–99, 109–115
Bundle of His, 26

cardiac output, 48, 84, 109
carotid sinus massage, 65
chaotic atrial tachycardia, 75
circus movement, 47
compensatory pause, 57–59
complete heart block. *See* atrioventricular block, third degree
coronary artery disease. *See* myocardial ischemia and infarction
coronary intensive care, 92

digitalis, 118, 144–156
    effects of, 144–146
    toxicity, 146–148
distortion of electrocardiogram. *See* artefact

ectopic rhythms, 45-91
electrical alternans, 121-122
electrocardiogram, incorrectly taken. *See* artefact
electrocardiographic measurements, 9-13
electrocardiography (principles of), 1-24
electrode placement, 15-18
enhanced automaticity, 47
escape beats, 30, 147, 148

fusion beats, 82-84, 161
   in Wolff-Parkinson-White syndrome, 136

"heart attack." *See* myocardial infarction
heart rate, measurement of, 9-10, 12
His-Purkinje system, 25-26
   in myocardial infarction, 109-115
hyperkalemia, 126-130
hypokalemia, 131, 152-156

idioventricular rhythm, 32, 43
   accelerated, 47, 82-84, 147
intraventricular block, 32-43
   in myocardial infarction, 109-115
isoproterenol, 118

J point, 4, 97
junctional premature beats, 52-52
junctional rhythms, 47, 75-80, 109, 147, 148, 151, 156

leads, electrocardiographic, 5-9
left anterior division (fascicle), 26, 38
   block of. *See* left anterior hemiblock
left anterior hemiblock, 38-42
left bundle branch, 26
left bundle branch block, 34-38
   atypical, 36-38
left posterior division (fascicle), 26, 40
   block of. *See* left posterior hemiblock
left posterior hemiblock, 40, 41-43, 113
lidocaine, 117, 118
Lown-Ganong-Levine syndrome, 136-138

measurements, electrocardiographic, 9-12
mitral valve, 1
multifocal atrial tachycardia, 75
myocardial infarction, 92-118
   arrhythmias in, 115-118
   artificial pacemakers in, 110-115
   conduction disorders in, 109-115
   electrocardiographic changes of, 93-94
   localization of, 97-109
   symptoms of, 93
myocardial ischemia, 94-97

nitroglycerine, 95
nonparoxysmal junctional tachycardia, 75-80, 147, 151

P wave, 3-4, 6, 25, 44-45
   and capture beats, 78-80
   and fusion beats, 82-84
   and ventricular premature beats, 54, 56-59
   in atrial premature beats, 48-51, 58
   in AV dissociation, 79-80, 86-87
   retrograde, in junctional rhythms, 51-52, 75
pacemakers, artificial, 28, 82, 157-170
   battery depletion, 165
   bipolar, 158
   component failure, 169
   demand (noncompetitive), 159-161
   exit block, 169
   fixed rate, 159
   follow-up of patients with, 165
   in myocardial infarction, 110-115, 118
   malfunction, 161-170
   pacing failure, 161-165
   principles of, 157-161
   sensing failure, 164-165
   stimulation threshold, 169
   temporary (external), 159, 166-170
   unipolar, 158
pericarditis, 119-122
potassium, 126-131, 152-156
preexcitation, 131-143
premature beats, 48-59. *See also* atrial, junctional and ventricular premature beats
Prinzmetal's angina, 97
procaineamide, 118, 131
propranolol, 118
pulmonary embolism, 122-126
pulmonary valve, 1
Purkinje cells, 26

Q wave (pathologic), 94
Q wave (septal), 6
QRS complex, 4, 6-8, 10-12
   mean frontal axis, 11-12
   See also specific conditions such as myocardial infarction
QT prolongation and ventricular arrhythmias, 131
quinidine, 118, 131

reentry, 47, 141-143
refractory period, 48-50
right bundle branch, 26
right bundle branch block, 33-34, 40-42, 113

sinoatrial arrest, 45, 147
sinoatrial block, 45, 147
sinoatrial node, 25, 146

sinus arrhythmia, 45
sinus bradycardia, 44
   in myocardial infarction, 117–118
sinus rhythm, 44
sinus tachycardia, 44
ST segment, 4, 93–94, 97, 119–126, 129–131, 146
standardization, 14
sudden death, 92, 165
supraventricular tachycardia, 59–82, 141–143
   in preexcitation, 138–141

T wave, 4, 93–94, 97, 126, 131, 146
tachycardia-bradycardia syndrome, 80–82
technical problems in electrocardiography, 13–24. *See also* artefact
thioridazine, 131
tricuspid valve, 1

trifascicular block, 40–43
   in myocardial infarction, 110

U wave, 4, 131

ventricular arrhythmias, 82–91
   caused by digitalis, 147
   in myocardial infarction, 115–118
   with QT prolongation, 131
ventricular fibrillation, 87–91
ventricular premature beats, 52–59, 69–75, 84, 91
ventricular tachycardia, 84–87
vulnerable period, 87–91

waves (electrocardiographic), 3–5
Wenckebach phenomenon, 27–28, 110, 148
Wolff-Parkinson-White syndrome, 134–136, 138–141